CW00494348

THE TRUTH ABOUT HYPERTENSION:

UNDERSTANDING THE CAUSES, SYMPTOMS, AND TREATMENT OF HIGH BLOOD PRESSURE

DR. MELISSA P. NELSON

1

TABLE OF CONTENTS

5

INTRODUCTION

The Truth About Hypertension: Understanding the Causes, Symptoms, and Treatment of High Blood Pressure is an essential guide that delves into the intricacies of one of the most prevalent health conditions in the world today. In this book, we will embark on a journey to unravel the mysteries surrounding high blood pressure, providing readers with a comprehensive understanding of its causes, symptoms, and various treatment options available.

Hypertension, commonly known as high blood pressure, affects millions of people worldwide and is a significant risk factor for serious health issues such as heart disease, stroke, and kidney problems. Despite its widespread impact, there is often confusion and misinformation surrounding this condition. Through this book, we aim to shed light on the truth about hypertension, equipping readers with the knowledge they need to navigate their own health journey effectively.

In the following chapters, we will explore the
multifaceted causes of hypertension, taking into
account both genetic predispositions and lifestyle
choices. By understanding the factors contributing to
high blood pressure, readers will gain insight into how
to minimize their risk and make informed decisions
regarding their health.

Recognizing the symptoms of hypertension is crucial
for early detection and intervention. In this book, we
will examine the common signs that indicate high blood
pressure, helping readers identify and seek medical
attention promptly. By doing so, individuals can take
control of their health and potentially prevent the onset
of complications.

Treatment options for hypertension encompass a wide
range of approaches, from lifestyle modifications to
medication. Through detailed explanations, we will
explore the importance of dietary choices, physical
activity, stress management, and other
non-pharmacological interventions. Additionally, we
will delve into the various types of antihypertensive

medications available, their mechanisms of action, and potential side effects. By presenting these treatment options, readers will be empowered to make informed decisions in consultation with their healthcare providers.

Throughout this book, we emphasize the significance of patient education and empowerment. Dispelling common misconceptions and presenting evidence-based information, we aim to equip readers with the tools needed to take control of their blood pressure and overall well-being. By understanding the truth about hypertension, individuals can proactively manage their health, reduce the risks associated with high blood pressure, and lead healthier, fulfilling lives.

"The Truth About Hypertension: Understanding the Causes, Symptoms, and Treatment of High Blood Pressure" is a comprehensive resource designed to provide clarity and guidance in the realm of hypertension. Whether you are someone living with high blood pressure, a caregiver, or simply interested in understanding this prevalent health condition, this book is a valuable tool to enhance your knowledge and empower you on your journey to optimal health.

CHAPTER 1

WHAT IS HYPERTENSION, AND WHY IS IT A HEALTH CONCERN?

Here are a few alternative definitions of hypertension:

1. Hypertension is a medical condition characterized by abnormally high blood pressure levels, which persistently exceed the normal range of 120/80 mmHg, potentially leading to increased risks of cardiovascular diseases.

2. Hypertension refers to a chronic health disorder characterized by elevated systemic arterial blood pressure, often resulting from a combination of genetic predisposition, unhealthy lifestyle choices, and underlying medical conditions.

3. Hypertension is a cardiovascular condition marked by consistently elevated blood pressure levels, exceeding the optimal range, that can strain the heart and damage

blood vessels, potentially leading to complications such
as heart attack, stroke, or kidney problems.

4. Hypertension, commonly known as high blood
pressure, is a condition in which the force exerted by
blood against the walls of arteries is chronically elevated,
posing a significant risk to overall cardiovascular health
and increasing the likelihood of developing severe
health issues.

5. Hypertension is a medical disorder characterized by a
persistent increase in blood pressure, exceeding the
normal range, which can impair the proper functioning
of vital organs, including the heart, brain, and kidneys,
if left uncontrolled.

It's important to note that while these definitions
convey the essence of hypertension, they may vary in
wording and emphasis. Hypertension is a complex
medical condition, and its understanding and treatment
should be guided by qualified healthcare professionals.

Why Is Hypertension A Health Concern?

Hypertension is a significant health concern due to its potential to cause serious complications and increase the risk of various cardiovascular diseases.

Here are some reasons why hypertension is a matter of concern:

1. Increased Risk of Heart Disease:

Hypertension forces the heart to work harder to pump blood throughout the body, leading to strain and enlargement of the heart muscle. Over time, this can contribute to the development of heart conditions such as coronary artery disease, heart failure, and heart attacks.

2. Higher Risk of Stroke:

High blood pressure damages and weakens the blood vessels, including those in the brain. This makes individuals with hypertension more susceptible to stroke, which occurs when the blood supply to the brain is interrupted or reduced. Strokes can result in significant disability or even be fatal.

3. Kidney Damage:

The kidneys play a crucial role in regulating blood pressure. Hypertension can impair kidney function and cause damage to the small blood vessels within the kidneys. Over time, this can lead to chronic kidney disease or kidney failure.

4. Increased Risk of Peripheral Artery Disease:

Hypertension can contribute to the development of peripheral artery disease, a condition characterized by narrowed arteries that reduce blood flow to the limbs, typically the legs. This can result in leg pain, difficulty walking, non-healing wounds, and, in severe cases, limb amputation.

5. Impact on Vision:

Uncontrolled hypertension can damage the blood vessels in the eyes, leading to vision problems or even vision loss. Hypertensive retinopathy is a condition where the blood vessels in the retina are affected, potentially causing blurred vision, bleeding in the eye, or complete loss of vision.

6. Other Health Complications:

Hypertension is associated with an increased risk of other health issues, including aneurysms (abnormal bulging of blood vessels), cognitive decline and dementia, sexual dysfunction, metabolic syndrome, and increased risk of developing diabetes.

It's crucial to note that hypertension often doesn't cause noticeable symptoms until it reaches an advanced stage or leads to a complication. Regular monitoring of blood pressure, lifestyle modifications, and appropriate medical management are essential to prevent or control hypertension and reduce the risk of associated health concerns.

CHAPTER 2

THE RISK FACTORS FOR DEVELOPING HYPERTENSION

Several risk factors contribute to the development of hypertension (high blood pressure). Understanding these risk factors can help individuals assess their likelihood of developing hypertension and take preventive measures.

Here are some key risk factors:

Age:

Advancing age is a significant risk factor for hypertension. As individuals get older, the risk of developing high blood pressure increases. This can be attributed to the natural aging process, which leads to a decrease in the elasticity of blood vessels, making them less efficient at regulating blood pressure.

Age is a well-established risk factor for developing hypertension (high blood pressure). As individuals grow older, the risk of hypertension increases. This phenomenon is commonly referred to as age-related or primary hypertension.

Several factors contribute to the age-related rise in blood pressure:

1. Arterial Stiffness: With age, the arteries tend to become less elastic and more rigid. This reduced elasticity makes it more difficult for the blood vessels to expand and contract effectively, resulting in higher blood pressure levels. Arterial stiffness is a natural consequence of aging and can contribute to the development of hypertension.

2. Decreased Renal Function: The kidneys play a vital role in regulating blood pressure by balancing sodium and fluid levels in the body. However, as individuals age, the kidneys may experience a decline in function. This can disrupt the body's ability to regulate

20

blood pressure effectively, leading to higher blood
pressure levels.

3. Hormonal Changes: Hormonal changes associated
with aging can impact blood pressure regulation. For
instance, as individuals age, hormone levels, such as
renin and aldosterone, may fluctuate. These hormones
play a role in maintaining fluid and electrolyte balance,
and their imbalances can contribute to hypertension.

4. Accumulated Effects of Other Risk Factors:
Over time, lifestyle choices and other risk factors can
accumulate and contribute to the development of
hypertension. Factors such as unhealthy diet, sedentary
lifestyle, obesity, and chronic stress may be more
prevalent as individuals age. These factors can
synergistically raise blood pressure, further increasing
the risk of hypertension.

It is important to note that while age is a significant risk
factor for developing hypertension, it does not mean
that hypertension is an inevitable consequence of aging.
Adopting a healthy lifestyle, including a balanced diet,

regular physical activity, stress management, maintaining a healthy weight, and avoiding tobacco and excessive alcohol use, can help mitigate the effects of aging on blood pressure.

Regular blood pressure monitoring is also crucial, especially as individuals age, to detect and manage hypertension early. With appropriate lifestyle modifications and, if necessary, medical interventions, individuals can effectively control their blood pressure and reduce the risk of hypertension-related complications, promoting overall cardiovascular health as they age.

Family History:

Having a family history of hypertension increases the risk of developing the condition. If your parents or close relatives have a history of high blood pressure, you may have a genetic predisposition to hypertension. Genetic factors can influence how the body regulates blood pressure, making some individuals more susceptible to developing hypertension.

Family history is considered a significant risk factor for developing hypertension (high blood pressure). If individuals have close family members, such as parents or siblings, who have been diagnosed with hypertension, their own risk of developing the condition increases.

Here's why family history plays a role in hypertension risk:

1. Genetic Predisposition: Genetic factors can influence an individual's susceptibility to hypertension. Certain genes can affect how the body regulates blood pressure and responds to various physiological factors. If individuals have a family history of hypertension, it suggests that they may have inherited genetic variations that make them more prone to developing the condition.

2. Shared Lifestyle and Environmental Factors: Families often share common lifestyles, dietary habits, and environmental exposures. These factors can contribute to hypertension risk. Unhealthy habits and behaviors, such as poor dietary choices, sedentary lifestyle, tobacco use, and excessive alcohol consumption, may be prevalent within families. When individuals grow up in such an environment, they are more likely to adopt similar habits, which can increase their risk of developing hypertension.

3. Cultural and Socioeconomic Influences: Family history of hypertension can also reflect shared cultural or socioeconomic influences. Certain ethnic or racial groups have a higher prevalence of hypertension, and individuals from these groups may have a greater risk due to both genetic and environmental factors. Socioeconomic factors such as limited access to healthcare, unhealthy living conditions, and stress associated with low socioeconomic status can also contribute to hypertension risk within families.

4. Awareness and Health Screening: Having a family member with hypertension may lead to increased awareness of the condition. Individuals who are aware of their family history may be more likely to monitor their blood pressure regularly and seek medical attention if needed. This awareness can promote early detection and management of hypertension, reducing the risk of complications.

While family history is a significant risk factor, it does not guarantee that individuals will develop hypertension. It serves as an indication that individuals may have an increased predisposition to the condition. By being aware of their family history, individuals can take proactive steps to prevent or manage hypertension. This includes adopting a healthy lifestyle, engaging in regular exercise, maintaining a balanced diet, managing stress, avoiding tobacco and excessive alcohol use, and seeking regular medical check-ups to monitor blood pressure levels. Early detection, lifestyle modifications, and appropriate medical interventions can help individuals with a family history of hypertension maintain optimal blood pressure and reduce the risk of related complications.

Unhealthy Diet:

Poor dietary choices play a significant role in the development of hypertension. Consuming a diet high in sodium (salt), saturated and trans fats, and low in essential nutrients like potassium, calcium, and magnesium can contribute to elevated blood pressure levels. Processed and fast foods, excessive salt intake, sugary beverages, and a lack of fruits and vegetables in the diet can increase the risk of hypertension.

An unhealthy diet is a significant risk factor for developing hypertension (high blood pressure). The foods we consume directly impact our blood pressure levels, and poor dietary choices can contribute to the development and progression of hypertension.

Here's how an unhealthy diet can increase the risk of hypertension:

1. High Sodium (Salt) Intake: Consuming excessive amounts of sodium is strongly linked to hypertension. A high-sodium diet disrupts the delicate balance of fluids in the body, leading to increased fluid retention and higher blood volume. This, in turn, raises blood pressure. Processed foods, fast food, canned soups, snacks, and condiments are often high in sodium. Limiting sodium intake by choosing fresh, minimally processed foods and avoiding adding extra salt to meals can help lower the risk of hypertension.

2. Low Potassium, Calcium, and Magnesium Intake: Adequate intake of minerals like potassium, calcium, and magnesium is essential for maintaining healthy blood pressure levels. Potassium helps relax blood vessel walls, while calcium and magnesium contribute to proper muscle function, including the muscles that control blood vessel tone. A diet lacking in these minerals may disrupt the balance and contribute to elevated blood pressure. To increase intake, individuals should include potassium-rich foods like bananas, leafy greens, citrus fruits, dairy products for

27

calcium, and nuts, seeds, and whole grains for magnesium.

3. Excessive Sugar and Added Sugars: A diet high in added sugars and sugary beverages can contribute to weight gain, obesity, and insulin resistance, all of which are risk factors for hypertension. Consuming excessive amounts of sugary drinks like soda, fruit juices, and sweetened beverages can lead to weight gain and metabolic disturbances that impact blood pressure regulation. Reducing the intake of sugary foods and drinks, opting for water or unsweetened alternatives, and choosing whole fruits instead of juices can help lower the risk of hypertension.

4. Low Fiber and High Fat Intake: A diet low in fiber and high in saturated and trans fats is associated with an increased risk of hypertension. Low-fiber diets can contribute to weight gain and obesity, while high intake of saturated and trans fats can lead to inflammation, arterial damage, and compromised blood pressure regulation. Opting for a diet rich in fruits, vegetables, whole grains, lean proteins, and healthy fats like those found in nuts, seeds, and olive oil can help lower the risk of hypertension.

5. Alcohol Consumption: Excessive alcohol consumption can contribute to high blood pressure. While moderate alcohol intake may have some cardiovascular benefits, excessive or heavy drinking can raise blood pressure levels and increase the risk of hypertension. To reduce the risk, it's recommended to consume alcohol in moderation, which means up to one drink per day for women and up to two drinks per day for men.

Adopting a healthy diet is crucial in preventing and managing hypertension. The Dietary Approaches to Stop Hypertension (DASH) eating plan, which emphasizes fruits, vegetables, whole grains, lean proteins, and low-fat dairy products while limiting sodium, added sugars, and unhealthy fats, has been shown to effectively lower blood pressure. Making conscious food choices, reading food labels, cooking at home, and seeking guidance from healthcare professionals or registered dietitians can help individuals modify their diet to reduce the risk of hypertension and promote overall cardiovascular health.

Sedentary Lifestyle:

Leading a sedentary lifestyle with little to no physical activity can increase the risk of hypertension. Lack of regular exercise and physical inactivity contribute to weight gain, obesity, and poor cardiovascular health, all of which can raise blood pressure levels. Engaging in regular aerobic exercise, such as brisk walking, jogging, swimming, or cycling, can help reduce the risk of developing hypertension.

A sedentary lifestyle is a significant risk factor for developing hypertension (high blood pressure). A sedentary lifestyle refers to a lack of regular physical activity or engaging in activities that involve minimal movement.

Here's how a sedentary lifestyle can contribute to the development of hypertension:

30

1. Weight Gain and Obesity: A sedentary lifestyle often leads to weight gain and obesity, both of which are known risk factors for hypertension. When individuals are inactive, they burn fewer calories, and unused calories can be stored as excess body weight. Excess weight puts additional strain on the heart and blood vessels, leading to increased blood pressure. Regular physical activity helps maintain a healthy weight and reduces the risk of hypertension.

2. Poor Cardiovascular Fitness: Lack of physical activity can lead to poor cardiovascular fitness. When individuals are sedentary, their heart and blood vessels become less efficient at pumping blood, leading to increased resistance in the arteries and higher blood pressure levels. Regular aerobic exercise improves cardiovascular fitness, strengthens the heart, and helps maintain healthy blood pressure.

3. Impaired Blood Vessel Function: Physical activity stimulates the production of nitric oxide, a compound that helps relax and dilate blood vessels. Inactivity, on

31

the other hand, can impair blood vessel function, leading to reduced flexibility and constriction of blood vessels. This constriction raises blood pressure levels and increases the workload on the heart. Regular exercise promotes healthy blood vessel function and helps keep blood pressure in check.

4. Insulin Resistance and Metabolic Disorders: A sedentary lifestyle is associated with insulin resistance and metabolic disorders like diabetes and metabolic syndrome. These conditions increase the risk of hypertension. Insulin resistance disrupts normal blood sugar regulation and can lead to higher blood pressure levels. Engaging in regular physical activity improves insulin sensitivity and helps manage these metabolic disorders, reducing the risk of hypertension.

5. Stress and Hormonal Imbalances: Sedentary lifestyles often contribute to increased stress levels, as physical activity is known to help alleviate stress. Chronic stress can trigger hormonal imbalances and lead to sustained elevated blood pressure. Regular exercise not only helps manage stress but also promotes

32

the release of endorphins, which are natural mood boosters that contribute to overall well-being.

To mitigate the risk of hypertension associated with a sedentary lifestyle, it's crucial to incorporate regular physical activity into daily routines. Engaging in aerobic exercises such as walking, jogging, swimming, cycling, or dancing for at least 150 minutes per week is recommended. Additionally, reducing sedentary behaviors like prolonged sitting and incorporating movement breaks throughout the day can help improve overall cardiovascular health and reduce the risk of hypertension. It's essential to find activities that are enjoyable and sustainable to maintain a physically active lifestyle in the long term. Consultation with healthcare professionals or fitness experts can provide personalized guidance on exercise routines and physical activity recommendations based on individual health status and goals.

Excess Weight and Obesity:

Being overweight or obese is a significant risk factor for hypertension. Excess body weight puts additional strain on the heart and blood vessels, leading to higher blood pressure. The accumulation of fat tissue can disrupt the normal functioning of hormones involved in blood pressure regulation. Maintaining a healthy weight through a balanced diet and regular physical activity is important in preventing hypertension.

Weight and obesity are significant risk factors for developing hypertension (high blood pressure). Excess body weight, particularly when it is concentrated around the waist area, puts additional strain on the heart and blood vessels, leading to increased blood pressure.

Here's how weight and obesity contribute to the development of hypertension:

1. Increased Blood Volume: Excess body weight requires an increased blood supply to provide oxygen and nutrients to the body's tissues. As a result, the heart has to pump more blood, which raises blood pressure.

34

The increased blood volume also puts a greater load on the blood vessels, causing them to become narrower and less flexible, further contributing to elevated blood pressure levels.

2. Insulin Resistance: Obesity is often associated with insulin resistance, a condition where cells become less responsive to the effects of insulin. Insulin resistance can lead to an increase in the production of insulin and higher levels of insulin in the blood. Elevated insulin levels can constrict blood vessels and promote sodium and fluid retention, leading to an increase in blood pressure.

3. Inflammatory Processes: Adipose tissue (fat cells) releases various substances known as adipokines, including inflammatory markers. In obese individuals, these adipokines are produced in higher amounts, leading to chronic low-grade inflammation. Inflammation can damage the inner lining of blood vessels and impair their ability to relax and constrict properly, resulting in elevated blood pressure.

4. Sleep Apnea: Obesity is strongly associated with sleep apnea, a sleep disorder characterized by interrupted breathing during sleep. Sleep apnea can lead to temporary increases in blood pressure during the night and reduced oxygen levels, which can contribute to hypertension. The combination of obesity and sleep apnea creates a vicious cycle, as sleep disturbances can further contribute to weight gain and obesity.

5. Hormonal Imbalances: Excess body fat can disrupt the normal balance of hormones involved in blood pressure regulation. Adipose tissue produces hormones that influence blood pressure, such as leptin and adiponectin. In obesity, these hormone levels may be altered, leading to impaired blood pressure control and increased risk of hypertension.

Addressing weight and obesity is crucial in preventing and managing hypertension. Weight loss through lifestyle modifications, including adopting a balanced and nutritious diet, increasing physical activity, and making sustainable behavior changes, can significantly reduce blood pressure levels. It is recommended to aim for a gradual and steady weight loss of about 1-2 pounds per week for long-term success.

In addition to weight loss, adopting a healthy lifestyle that includes regular physical activity, managing stress, avoiding tobacco and excessive alcohol use, and maintaining a balanced diet low in sodium and high in fruits, vegetables, whole grains, lean proteins, and healthy fats, can help lower the risk of hypertension. Monitoring blood pressure regularly and seeking guidance from healthcare professionals or registered dietitians can provide personalized recommendations for weight management and overall cardiovascular health.

Tobacco and Alcohol Use:

Tobacco use, both smoking and smokeless tobacco, significantly increases the risk of hypertension. Chemicals in tobacco products can damage blood vessels, promote inflammation, and contribute to the development of hypertension. Excessive alcohol consumption can also raise blood pressure levels and

contribute to weight gain. It's important to avoid
tobacco use and moderate alcohol intake to reduce the
risk of hypertension.

Tobacco and alcohol use are significant risk factors for
developing hypertension (high blood pressure). Both
smoking and excessive alcohol consumption can have
detrimental effects on cardiovascular health and
contribute to the development and progression of
hypertension.

Here's how tobacco and alcohol use increase the risk of hypertension:

1. Smoking and Nicotine: Tobacco smoke contains
numerous chemicals that can damage blood vessels and
interfere with normal blood flow. Nicotine, a highly
addictive substance present in cigarettes, causes blood
vessels to constrict and raises blood pressure
temporarily. Chronic smoking leads to sustained
elevation in blood pressure, as well as increased heart
rate and reduced oxygen supply to the tissues.

Prolonged exposure to tobacco smoke and nicotine can contribute to the development of hypertension.

2. Arterial Stiffness: Smoking has been linked to increased arterial stiffness, which is a significant risk factor for hypertension. Arterial stiffness reduces the ability of blood vessels to expand and contract effectively, resulting in higher blood pressure levels. Long-term smoking can lead to structural changes in blood vessels, compromising their elasticity and promoting hypertension.

3. Alcohol and Blood Pressure: While moderate alcohol consumption may have some cardiovascular benefits, excessive or heavy drinking can raise blood pressure levels. Alcohol is a vasodilator, meaning it relaxes and widens blood vessels. However, excessive alcohol intake can disrupt this balance and lead to sustained high blood pressure. Alcohol also stimulates the release of stress hormones, which can constrict blood vessels and elevate blood pressure.

4. Weight Gain and Obesity: Both tobacco and alcohol use have been associated with weight gain and obesity, which are independent risk factors for hypertension. Smoking cessation can lead to weight gain in some individuals, while excessive alcohol consumption can contribute to calorie intake and promote weight gain. The excess body weight puts additional strain on the heart and blood vessels, leading to increased blood pressure.

5. Interactions with Medications: Smoking and excessive alcohol use can interfere with the effectiveness of certain medications used to treat hypertension. For example, smoking reduces the efficacy of antihypertensive medications and may require higher doses to achieve blood pressure control. Alcohol consumption can also interact with certain medications and reduce their effectiveness or increase side effects.

To reduce the risk of hypertension associated with tobacco and alcohol use, it is essential to adopt healthy habits:

- Quit smoking: Smoking cessation is one of the most important steps individuals can take to improve their cardiovascular health. Quitting smoking not only reduces the risk of hypertension but also lowers the risk of heart disease, stroke, and other serious health conditions.

- Limit alcohol consumption: Moderate alcohol intake is defined as up to one drink per day for women and up to two drinks per day for men. It's important to consume alcohol in moderation and be aware of its potential effects on blood pressure. For individuals with hypertension or those at risk, it may be advisable to further limit alcohol consumption or avoid it altogether.

- Seek support: Quitting smoking or reducing alcohol consumption can be challenging. Seeking support from healthcare professionals, counseling services, support groups, or helplines can provide valuable guidance, resources, and encouragement.

By eliminating tobacco use, moderating alcohol consumption, and adopting a healthy lifestyle that includes regular physical activity, a balanced diet, stress management, and weight control, individuals can significantly reduce the risk of hypertension and promote overall cardiovascular health. Regular blood pressure monitoring and consultation with healthcare professionals are essential for managing and preventing hypertension.

Stress:

Chronic stress and high levels of psychological stress can contribute to the development of hypertension. When stressed, the body releases stress hormones that temporarily increase blood pressure. Prolonged or frequent stress can lead to sustained elevated blood pressure levels. Managing stress through techniques like exercise, relaxation exercises, mindfulness, and adopting healthy coping mechanisms is important for maintaining healthy blood pressure.

Stress is recognized as a risk factor for developing hypertension (high blood pressure). While stress itself may not directly cause hypertension, it can contribute to the development and exacerbation of the condition.

Here's how chronic stress can increase the risk of hypertension:

1. Increased Sympathetic Nervous System Activity: When individuals experience stress, their body's sympathetic nervous system is activated, leading to the release of stress hormones such as adrenaline and cortisol. These hormones temporarily raise blood pressure by constricting blood vessels and increasing heart rate. Prolonged or chronic stress can result in sustained elevation of blood pressure, contributing to the development of hypertension.

2. Unhealthy Coping Mechanisms: When faced with stress, individuals may adopt unhealthy coping mechanisms such as overeating, physical inactivity, excessive alcohol consumption, or tobacco use. These behaviors can directly contribute to the development of

hypertension. For example, overeating unhealthy foods can lead to weight gain, while physical inactivity can contribute to weight gain and reduced cardiovascular fitness.

3. Disrupted Stress Hormone Regulation: Chronic stress can disrupt the normal regulation of stress hormones in the body. Prolonged elevation of cortisol levels can affect blood pressure regulation mechanisms, leading to increased sodium and water retention, reduced nitric oxide production (which helps relax blood vessels), and elevated blood pressure levels.

4. Emotional Factors: Stress can also impact emotional well-being and mental health. Anxiety, depression, and chronic psychological stress have been associated with an increased risk of hypertension. Emotional factors may contribute to unhealthy lifestyle behaviors, poor adherence to medication regimens, and physiological changes that can affect blood pressure.

5. Sleep Disturbances: Chronic stress can disrupt sleep patterns, leading to inadequate sleep or poor quality sleep. Sleep deprivation or poor sleep quality has been linked to elevated blood pressure and an increased risk of developing hypertension.

Managing stress is crucial in preventing and managing hypertension.

Here are some strategies to help reduce stress levels:

1. Stress Management Techniques: Engaging in stress-reducing activities such as deep breathing exercises, meditation, yoga, mindfulness, or engaging in hobbies can help lower stress levels.

2. Regular Physical Activity: Regular exercise can help reduce stress by promoting the release of endorphins, improving mood, and enhancing overall well-being. Aim for at least 150 minutes of moderate-intensity aerobic exercise per week.

3. Healthy Lifestyle Choices: Adopting a healthy lifestyle that includes a balanced diet, limiting alcohol consumption, avoiding tobacco use, and getting enough sleep can help manage stress and reduce the risk of hypertension.

4. Social Support: Building and maintaining strong social connections can provide emotional support, help cope with stress, and promote overall well-being.

5. Seeking Professional Help: If stress becomes overwhelming or persists despite efforts to manage it, seeking help from mental health professionals, therapists, or counselors can provide guidance and support in developing effective coping strategies.

While it may not be possible to eliminate all sources of stress, managing stress effectively is essential for overall health and well-being. By implementing stress reduction techniques and adopting a healthy lifestyle, individuals can help reduce the risk of hypertension and promote cardiovascular health. Regular blood pressure monitoring and consultation with healthcare professionals are important for managing and preventing hypertension.

Underlying Medical Conditions:

Certain medical conditions increase the risk of hypertension. These include diabetes, kidney disease, sleep apnea, hormone disorders (such as Cushing's syndrome or hyperthyroidism), and certain chronic conditions like high cholesterol or cardiovascular disease. Proper management and treatment of these underlying conditions are crucial in preventing or controlling hypertension.

Underlying medical conditions can be significant risk factors for developing hypertension (high blood pressure). Certain health conditions can directly contribute to the development or exacerbation of hypertension.

Here are some examples of underlying medical conditions that increase the risk of hypertension:

1. Kidney Disease: The kidneys play a crucial role in regulating blood pressure by balancing fluids and

47

electrolytes in the body. When kidney function is impaired due to conditions like chronic kidney disease or renal artery stenosis (narrowing of the arteries supplying blood to the kidneys), it can lead to increased fluid retention and elevated blood pressure.

2. Endocrine Disorders: Hormonal imbalances caused by endocrine disorders can contribute to hypertension. Conditions such as Cushing's syndrome (excess cortisol production), primary aldosteronism (excess aldosterone production), and pheochromocytoma (tumor in the adrenal glands) can lead to elevated blood pressure levels.

3. Thyroid Disorders: Both an underactive thyroid (hypothyroidism) and an overactive thyroid (hyperthyroidism) can impact blood pressure regulation. Hypothyroidism can cause a decrease in heart rate and cardiac output, leading to elevated blood pressure. Hyperthyroidism, on the other hand, can increase heart rate and cardiac output, potentially resulting in hypertension.

4. Diabetes: People with diabetes, especially type 2 diabetes, are at an increased risk of developing hypertension. The combination of insulin resistance, abnormal blood sugar control, and metabolic changes associated with diabetes can contribute to the development of high blood pressure.

5. Sleep Apnea: Sleep apnea is a sleep disorder characterized by interrupted breathing during sleep. It has been linked to hypertension due to the intermittent drops in oxygen levels and increased stress responses during sleep. The combination of sleep apnea and hypertension can create a cycle, as hypertension can also worsen sleep apnea.

6. Cardiovascular Conditions: Certain cardiovascular conditions, such as heart disease, heart failure, and atherosclerosis (hardening of the arteries), can increase the risk of hypertension. These conditions can disrupt normal blood flow, increase the workload on the heart, and contribute to elevated blood pressure.

7. Adrenal Disorders: Adrenal disorders, such as adrenal tumors or adrenal gland dysfunction, can result in the overproduction of hormones that regulate blood pressure. Excessive production of aldosterone or catecholamines can lead to hypertension.

Managing underlying medical conditions is essential in preventing and controlling hypertension. Treatment strategies may involve a combination of lifestyle modifications, medications, and targeted therapies to address the specific medical condition. It is important to work closely with healthcare professionals to develop a comprehensive management plan that includes regular monitoring of blood pressure and adherence to treatment recommendations.

In addition to managing the underlying medical condition, adopting a healthy lifestyle is crucial in managing hypertension. This includes maintaining a balanced diet, engaging in regular physical activity, managing stress, limiting alcohol consumption, avoiding tobacco use, and maintaining a healthy weight.

By addressing and effectively managing underlying medical conditions and adopting a holistic approach to cardiovascular health, individuals can reduce the risk of hypertension and promote overall well-being. Regular check-ups and open communication with healthcare professionals are essential in managing and preventing hypertension in the presence of underlying medical conditions.

While these risk factors contribute to the development of hypertension, it's important to note that lifestyle modifications, such as adopting a healthy diet, engaging in regular physical activity, managing stress, maintaining a healthy weight, avoiding tobacco and excessive alcohol use, can significantly reduce the risk or help manage hypertension effectively. Regular blood pressure monitoring and seeking appropriate medical care are essential for early detection and management of hypertension.

CHAPTER 3

THE SYMPTOMS OF HYPERTENSION AND HOW THEY CAN BE RECOGNIZED AND DIAGNOSED.

Hypertension, commonly known as high blood pressure, is often referred to as a "silent killer" because it typically does not cause noticeable symptoms in its early stages. Most people with hypertension do not experience any specific symptoms, which is why it is essential to regularly monitor blood pressure levels. However, as hypertension progresses or if blood pressure levels become severely elevated, some individuals may experience certain symptoms or signs that could indicate the presence of hypertension or its complications.

Here are some possible symptoms of hypertension:

Headaches:
Persistent or recurring headaches, particularly in the morning, can be a symptom of hypertension. However,

headaches alone are not specific to hypertension and
can be caused by various factors. It is important to note
that not all individuals with high blood pressure
experience headaches.

Blurred Vision:

In some cases, hypertension can lead to changes in
vision or blurred vision. This can occur if high blood
pressure affects the blood vessels in the eyes. However,
vision changes can also be caused by other conditions,
so it is important to consult a healthcare professional
for proper evaluation.

Dizziness or Vertigo:

Feeling lightheaded, dizzy, or experiencing episodes of
vertigo (a spinning sensation) can occasionally be
associated with hypertension, especially if blood
pressure levels are significantly elevated. However, there
are many other potential causes for these symptoms, so
a thorough evaluation is necessary to determine the
underlying cause.

Chest Pain:

Chest pain or discomfort may occur in individuals with hypertension, particularly if it leads to heart-related complications such as angina (reduced blood flow to the heart) or heart attack. However, chest pain can have various causes, and not all cases are related to hypertension.

It is important to note that these symptoms are not exclusive to hypertension and can be associated with other health conditions as well. Additionally, many people with hypertension do not experience any noticeable symptoms, which is why regular blood pressure monitoring is crucial in identifying and managing the condition.

If you experience any of these symptoms or have concerns about your blood pressure, it is recommended to consult a healthcare professional for proper evaluation and diagnosis. Regular check-ups and blood pressure measurements are essential in detecting and managing hypertension. Early detection and appropriate treatment can help prevent complications and maintain cardiovascular health.

ways to recognize the symptoms of hypertension

Regular Blood Pressure Monitoring:

The most reliable way to recognize hypertension is through regular blood pressure monitoring. Blood pressure is measured using two numbers: systolic pressure (the top number) and diastolic pressure (the bottom number). A blood pressure reading of 120/80 mmHg is considered normal. Readings consistently above 130/80 mmHg or higher may indicate hypertension. It is important to measure blood pressure regularly, especially as you age or if you have risk factors for hypertension.

Elevated Blood Pressure Readings:

If you measure your blood pressure and consistently find readings above the normal range, it may be an indication of hypertension. It is essential to measure blood pressure correctly, using a validated blood

pressure cuff, following the proper technique, and
ensuring a calm and relaxed state.

Awareness of Risk Factors:

Understanding the risk factors associated with
hypertension can help in recognizing its potential
symptoms. Risk factors include advancing age, family
history of hypertension, obesity or overweight,
sedentary lifestyle, unhealthy diet (high in salt, saturated
fats, and processed foods), tobacco and alcohol use,
chronic stress, certain medical conditions (such as
kidney disease or diabetes), and certain medications
(such as oral contraceptives or nonsteroidal
anti-inflammatory drugs). If you have one or more of
these risk factors, it is important to be vigilant and
monitor your blood pressure regularly.

Presence of Complications:

In some cases, hypertension can lead to complications
that may present with symptoms. These complications
include heart disease, heart failure, stroke, kidney
problems, and eye damage. Symptoms related to these
complications may include chest pain, shortness of

breath, irregular heartbeat, difficulty speaking or understanding speech, sudden severe headache, vision changes, and swelling of the ankles or legs. If you experience any of these symptoms, it is important to seek immediate medical attention.

It is important to note that hypertension is a chronic condition that often develops gradually over time. Many people with hypertension may not experience any noticeable symptoms. Regular blood pressure monitoring, routine check-ups with a healthcare professional, and adopting a healthy lifestyle are crucial in recognizing and managing hypertension. If you have concerns about your blood pressure or are at risk for hypertension, it is recommended to consult a healthcare professional for proper evaluation and guidance.

Diagnosing hypertension

Typically, this involves a combination of blood pressure measurements and an evaluation of potential symptoms or complications. Since hypertension often does not present noticeable symptoms, the primary method of diagnosis is through blood pressure monitoring.

Here are the steps involved in diagnosing hypertension:

Blood Pressure Measurement:

Blood pressure is measured using a blood pressure cuff and a sphygmomanometer or an automated device. It is important to measure blood pressure correctly and follow standardized guidelines. The measurement includes two numbers: systolic pressure (the top number) and diastolic pressure (the bottom number). A normal blood pressure reading is typically around 120/80 mmHg.

Multiple Readings:

A single blood pressure reading may not be sufficient to diagnose hypertension. Multiple blood pressure readings are taken on separate occasions to confirm the presence of sustained high blood pressure. These readings should be taken at different times of the day and in a relaxed state. Ideally, blood pressure should be measured on several occasions over a period of time, such as several weeks or months, to establish a pattern.

Ambulatory Blood Pressure Monitoring:

In some cases, healthcare professionals may recommend ambulatory blood pressure monitoring. This involves wearing a portable blood pressure monitoring device that automatically measures blood pressure at regular intervals over a 24-hour period. This method provides a more comprehensive assessment of blood pressure patterns throughout the day and night, reducing the potential influence of "white coat hypertension" (elevated blood pressure in a clinical setting).

Evaluation of Symptoms and Complications:

While hypertension often does not cause noticeable symptoms, healthcare professionals may inquire about any symptoms or complications that may be related to high blood pressure. Symptoms such as persistent headaches, vision changes, chest pain, shortness of breath, or signs of complications like heart disease or kidney problems may prompt further investigation and evaluation.

Additional Diagnostic Tests:

In some cases, healthcare professionals may recommend additional tests to evaluate organ damage or identify any underlying causes contributing to hypertension. These tests may include blood tests to assess kidney function, cholesterol levels, and blood glucose levels. Other diagnostic imaging tests, such as echocardiograms or ultrasounds, may be performed to evaluate the heart, blood vessels, and other organs.

It is important to work closely with a healthcare professional for an accurate diagnosis of hypertension. Regular blood pressure monitoring, routine check-ups, and open communication with healthcare professionals are crucial in diagnosing and managing hypertension effectively. Early detection and appropriate treatment can help prevent complications and maintain cardiovascular health.

CHAPTER 4

HOW HYPERTENSION IS MEASURED

Hypertension, or high blood pressure, is measured using a blood pressure cuff and a sphygmomanometer or an automated device. The measurement involves determining two numbers: systolic pressure and diastolic pressure.

Here is a step-by-step guide on how hypertension is measured:

Prepare the Equipment:
Ensure that you have the necessary equipment, including a blood pressure cuff, a sphygmomanometer (an instrument used to measure blood pressure), and a stethoscope (for manual measurements). If using an automated device, make sure it is properly calibrated and functioning.

Positioning:

Sit in a chair with your back supported, feet flat on the
ground, and arm comfortably resting on a flat surface.
The arm being used for the measurement should be
bare, with no clothing constricting the upper arm.

Wrapping the Cuff:

Wrap the blood pressure cuff around the upper arm,
just above the elbow. The cuff should fit snugly but not
be too tight or loose. Ensure that the cuff's lower edge is
about 2-3 centimeters above the bend of the elbow.

Identifying the Brachial Artery:

Locate the brachial artery on the inside of the arm,
slightly below the cuff's lower edge. This is the artery
that will be compressed and released during the
measurement.

Inflating the Cuff:

 Inflate the cuff by squeezing the bulb or pressing the
appropriate button on the automated device. The cuff
should inflate to a pressure above the expected systolic
pressure, typically around 180 mmHg.

Deflating the Cuff:

Gradually release the pressure in the cuff. If using a
manual sphygmomanometer, listen for the first tapping
sound (Korotkoff sound) with the stethoscope over the
brachial artery as the pressure decreases. If using an
automated device, it will display the readings.

Recording the Measurements:

Note the two numbers displayed or listen for the
sounds if using a manual sphygmomanometer. The first
sound indicates the systolic pressure, and the
disappearance of sound indicates the diastolic pressure.
Record the readings in millimeters of mercury
(mmHg).

Repeat and Average:

For accuracy, it is recommended to take multiple blood
pressure readings at different times on separate
occasions. This helps account for variations and ensures
a more reliable measurement. Take at least two readings,
ideally with a gap of a few minutes, and calculate the
average of the results.

Interpreting the Measurements:

Blood pressure is typically expressed as a ratio of systolic pressure over diastolic pressure (e.g., 120/80 mmHg). Normal blood pressure is considered to be around 120/80 mmHg. Elevated blood pressure is defined as readings consistently above 130/80 mmHg, which may indicate hypertension.

It is important to note that blood pressure measurements may vary throughout the day due to factors such as physical activity, stress, and time of day. Regular blood pressure monitoring and consultation with a healthcare professional are crucial in determining accurate blood pressure levels and diagnosing hypertension.

Blood Pressure Reading

Blood pressure readings provide information about the force of blood against the walls of the arteries. A blood pressure measurement consists of two numbers: systolic pressure and diastolic pressure. These numbers are expressed in millimeters of mercury (mmHg). Here's what each number represents and how to interpret blood pressure readings:

Systolic Pressure:
The top number in a blood pressure reading represents the systolic pressure. It indicates the pressure in the arteries when the heart contracts and pumps blood out. This phase is known as systole. A normal systolic pressure is typically below 120 mmHg.

Diastolic Pressure:
The bottom number in a blood pressure reading represents the diastolic pressure. It indicates the pressure in the arteries when the heart is at rest and filling with blood between beats. This phase is known as diastole. A normal diastolic pressure is typically below 80 mmHg.

Interpreting Blood Pressure Readings:

- Normal Blood Pressure:

A normal blood pressure reading is typically around 120/80 mmHg or lower. This indicates that blood pressure is within a healthy range, and there is no immediate concern for hypertension.

- Elevated Blood Pressure:

Elevated blood pressure is defined as systolic pressure ranging from 120 to 129 mmHg and diastolic pressure below 80 mmHg. It is a warning sign that blood pressure is higher than ideal, and lifestyle modifications may be recommended to prevent the development of hypertension.

Hypertension

- Stage 1 Hypertension:

Stage 1 hypertension is indicated by systolic pressure ranging from 130 to 139 mmHg or diastolic pressure ranging from 80 to 89 mmHg. This stage suggests the presence of mild hypertension and may require lifestyle changes and, in some cases, medication.

- Stage 2 Hypertension:

Stage 2 hypertension is indicated by systolic pressure of 140 mmHg or higher or diastolic pressure of 90 mmHg or higher. This stage suggests the presence of moderate to severe hypertension and typically requires a combination of lifestyle modifications and medication to manage blood pressure effectively.

- Hypertensive Crisis:

A hypertensive crisis occurs when blood pressure readings reach 180/120 mmHg or higher. This is a severe condition that requires immediate medical attention, as it can lead to organ damage and life-threatening complications.

It is important to note that a diagnosis of hypertension is not made based on a single blood pressure reading. Multiple readings taken on separate occasions are needed to confirm the presence of sustained high blood pressure. Blood pressure can vary throughout the day due to factors such as physical activity, stress, and time of day. Regular blood pressure monitoring and consultation with a healthcare professional are essential in interpreting and managing blood pressure readings accurately.

Testing Blood Pressure

There are several methods available for testing blood pressure, each offering different approaches to measuring and monitoring blood pressure levels. Here are some common blood pressure testing methods:

Manual or Auscultatory Method:
This traditional method involves using a sphygmomanometer, a cuff, and a stethoscope. The cuff is wrapped around the upper arm, and the healthcare professional inflates it to temporarily cut off blood flow. They then gradually release the pressure while listening to the sounds of blood flow using the stethoscope placed over the brachial artery. The first sound heard (Korotkoff sound) indicates the systolic pressure, and the point where the sound disappears indicates the diastolic pressure. This method requires training and expertise to accurately measure blood pressure.

Automated Method:

Automated blood pressure monitors are widely used
and provide a convenient way to measure blood
pressure at home or in clinical settings. These devices
usually consist of an electronic unit and a cuff. The cuff
is wrapped around the upper arm, and the device
automatically inflates and deflates the cuff to measure
blood pressure. The readings are displayed digitally on
the device. Automated monitors may use oscillometry
or another technology to detect blood flow and
calculate blood pressure.

Ambulatory Blood Pressure Monitoring (ABPM):

ABPM involves wearing a portable blood pressure
monitor that automatically measures blood pressure at
regular intervals throughout the day and night,
typically over a 24-hour period. The monitor is
typically worn on the upper arm and is connected to a
cuff. It inflates and deflates the cuff periodically to
obtain blood pressure readings. ABPM provides a
comprehensive assessment of blood pressure patterns
during daily activities and sleep, reducing the influence

of "white coat hypertension" (elevated blood pressure in
a clinical setting).

Home Blood Pressure Monitoring:

Home blood pressure monitoring involves using an
automated blood pressure monitor to measure blood
pressure at home. This method allows individuals to
monitor their blood pressure regularly, providing
valuable information for healthcare professionals to
assess blood pressure trends and adjust treatment plans.
It is important to use a validated device, follow the
manufacturer's instructions, and maintain a log of
readings to share with healthcare professionals.

Regardless of the method used, it is important to follow
guidelines for proper blood pressure measurement,
including being in a relaxed state, avoiding caffeine or
smoking beforehand, and using the appropriate cuff
size for accurate results. Regular blood pressure
monitoring, whether done at home or in a clinical
setting, is crucial for managing hypertension and
assessing the effectiveness of treatment. It is
recommended to consult a healthcare professional for

guidance on the most suitable blood pressure testing method and how to interpret the results accurately.

CHAPTER 5

THE TYPES OF HYPERTENSION

Hypertension, or high blood pressure, can be classified into two main types: primary (essential) hypertension and secondary hypertension.

Let's explore each type in more detail:

Primary Hypertension:

Primary hypertension, also known as essential hypertension, is the most common type of high blood pressure, accounting for approximately 90-95% of all cases. It is called "primary" or "essential" because it typically develops gradually over time without a specific identifiable cause. Instead, it is believed to result from a complex interplay of genetic, environmental, and lifestyle factors.

Here are key points about primary hypertension:

Risk Factors:

Primary hypertension is influenced by various risk factors, including:

- **Age:** The risk of developing hypertension increases with age.

- **Family History**: Having a family history of hypertension increases the likelihood of developing the condition.

- **Obesity:** Excess weight and obesity are significant risk factors for primary hypertension.

- **Unhealthy Diet:** A diet high in sodium (salt), saturated fats, and cholesterol can contribute to high blood pressure.

- **Sedentary Lifestyle:** Lack of physical activity and leading a sedentary lifestyle increase the risk of hypertension.

- **Tobacco and Alcohol Use**: Smoking and excessive alcohol consumption can raise blood pressure.

- **Chronic Stress:** Persistent stress or long-term exposure to stressful situations can impact blood pressure levels.

Progression and Symptoms:

 Primary hypertension often develops gradually over
many years. In its early stages, it may be asymptomatic
or present with mild, nonspecific symptoms that can
easily go unnoticed. Symptoms may manifest later as
blood pressure continues to rise, and they can include
headaches, dizziness, shortness of breath, chest pain,
fatigue, and visual changes. However, it's important to
note that many people with primary hypertension may
not experience any symptoms until it reaches an
advanced stage or causes complications.

Diagnosis:

Primary hypertension is diagnosed based on blood
pressure measurements. Multiple readings taken on
separate occasions are needed to confirm the presence of
sustained high blood pressure. The American Heart
Association (AHA) defines hypertension as a blood
pressure reading consistently at or above 130/80
mmHg. Regular blood pressure monitoring by a
healthcare professional is crucial for accurate diagnosis
and management.

Management:

The management of primary hypertension primarily involves lifestyle modifications and, in some cases, medication. Lifestyle changes may include:

- Adopting a healthy diet rich in fruits, vegetables, whole grains, and lean proteins while limiting sodium and saturated fats.

- Engaging in regular physical activity, aiming for at least 150 minutes of moderate-intensity aerobic exercise per week.

- Maintaining a healthy weight or losing weight if overweight or obese.

- Limiting alcohol consumption and avoiding tobacco use.

- Managing stress through relaxation techniques, exercise, or counseling.

In cases where lifestyle modifications alone are insufficient to control blood pressure, healthcare professionals may prescribe antihypertensive medications. These medications work to lower blood pressure and reduce the risk of complications associated with hypertension.

It is important for individuals with primary hypertension to have regular check-ups, monitor their blood pressure at home if advised by their healthcare provider, and comply with the recommended treatment plan. By managing blood pressure effectively, individuals with primary hypertension can reduce the risk of cardiovascular disease and other complications.

Secondary Hypertension:
Secondary hypertension refers to high blood pressure that is caused by an identifiable underlying medical condition or specific factors. Unlike primary hypertension, which is the most common form and has no specific cause, secondary hypertension can be attributed to various factors and health conditions.

Here are important points about secondary hypertension:

Underlying Medical Conditions:
Secondary hypertension can be associated with several underlying medical conditions, including:

- **Kidney Problems:** Conditions such as chronic kidney disease, renal artery stenosis, or polycystic kidney disease can lead to hypertension.

- **Hormonal Disorders:** Certain hormonal imbalances, such as primary aldosteronism (Conn's syndrome), Cushing's syndrome, or pheochromocytoma (a tumor in the adrenal glands), can cause high blood pressure.

- **Medications and Substances:** Some medications, such as nonsteroidal anti-inflammatory drugs (NSAIDs), oral contraceptives, and certain antidepressants, as well as substances like alcohol and illicit drugs, can contribute to hypertension.

- **Sleep Apnea:** Obstructive sleep apnea, a sleep disorder characterized by breathing interruptions during sleep, is associated with hypertension.

- **Endocrine Disorders:** Conditions like hyperthyroidism or hypothyroidism, as well as disorders affecting the adrenal glands, can lead to secondary hypertension.

- **Coarctation of the Aorta**: A congenital heart defect where the main artery (aorta) is narrowed, causing high blood pressure in the arms but low blood pressure in the legs.

- **Pregnancy-Induced Hypertension:** Gestational hypertension or preeclampsia, a condition that occurs during pregnancy, can cause high blood pressure.

- **Other Factors:** Certain cancers, certain autoimmune diseases, and the use of certain medications or substances can contribute to secondary hypertension.

Diagnosis:

Identifying the underlying cause of secondary hypertension is essential for effective management. Healthcare professionals may perform various tests and evaluations, including blood tests, urine tests, imaging studies, hormone level assessments, and specialized tests to identify specific conditions.

Management:

The management of secondary hypertension involves addressing the underlying cause while also controlling high blood pressure. Treatment strategies may include:

- Treating Underlying Medical Conditions:
Managing the specific medical condition causing
hypertension, such as kidney disease, hormonal
disorders, or sleep apnea.

- Medication Adjustment: Assessing and adjusting
medications that may be contributing to high blood
pressure.

- Lifestyle Modifications: Adopting lifestyle
changes similar to those recommended for primary
hypertension, including a healthy diet, regular exercise,
stress management, and avoiding tobacco and excessive
alcohol use.

- Medication for Blood Pressure Control:
Antihypertensive medications may be prescribed to
help lower blood pressure and manage hypertension
effectively.

Prognosis:
The prognosis for secondary hypertension depends on
the underlying cause and the success of managing both
the condition causing hypertension and blood pressure
levels. With proper diagnosis, treatment, and blood
pressure control, many individuals with secondary

hypertension can achieve normal or near-normal blood pressure levels and reduce the risk of complications.

It is crucial to work closely with healthcare professionals to identify and manage the underlying cause of secondary hypertension. Regular blood pressure monitoring, adherence to prescribed medications, and necessary lifestyle modifications are important for long-term management and reducing the risk of complications associated with hypertension.

CHAPTER 6

THE CAUSES OF HYPERTENSION

Hypertension, or high blood pressure, can have various causes, including both modifiable and non-modifiable factors. Understanding the underlying causes is important for effective management and prevention.

Here are some key causes of hypertension:

Modifiable Causes:

- Unhealthy Lifestyle:
Certain lifestyle factors can contribute to the development of hypertension. These include a poor diet high in sodium (salt), saturated fats, and cholesterol, as well as excessive alcohol consumption, tobacco use, and physical inactivity.

- Obesity:
Excess body weight, particularly abdominal obesity, is strongly associated with an increased risk of

81

hypertension. The extra weight puts additional strain on the heart and blood vessels, leading to elevated blood pressure.

- High Sodium Intake:

Consuming too much sodium in the diet can lead to fluid retention and increased blood volume, causing blood pressure to rise. Processed foods, fast foods, and excessive salt usage are common sources of high sodium intake.

- Sedentary Lifestyle:

Lack of regular physical activity and leading a sedentary lifestyle can contribute to the development of hypertension. Regular exercise helps maintain cardiovascular health and promotes normal blood pressure.

- Stress:

Chronic stress can play a role in the development and exacerbation of hypertension. Stress activates the body's "fight or flight" response, which can raise blood pressure temporarily. Prolonged stress can lead to sustained high blood pressure.

Non-Modifiable Causes:

- Age:
As individuals age, the risk of developing hypertension increases. This is primarily due to age-related changes in blood vessels and the reduced elasticity of arterial walls.

- Family History:
Having a family history of hypertension increases the risk of developing the condition. Genetic factors can influence blood pressure regulation and contribute to familial patterns of hypertension.

- Ethnicity:
Certain ethnic groups, such as African-Americans, have a higher prevalence of hypertension. This increased susceptibility may be attributed to genetic and environmental factors.

- Gender:

Hypertension is more common in men compared to premenopausal women. However, after menopause, the risk for women increases and becomes similar to that of men.

- Underlying Medical Conditions:

Various medical conditions and diseases can contribute to the development of hypertension. These include chronic kidney disease, hormonal disorders (e.g., primary aldosteronism), thyroid disorders, adrenal gland disorders, coarctation of the aorta, and sleep apnea.

- Medications and Substances:

Certain medications, such as nonsteroidal anti-inflammatory drugs (NSAIDs), oral contraceptives, decongestants, and some antidepressants, as well as substances like alcohol and illicit drugs, can raise blood pressure.

It is important to note that in many cases, hypertension develops due to a combination of multiple factors. Individuals with hypertension often have a combination of genetic predisposition, lifestyle-related causes, and other contributing factors. It is advisable to consult with a healthcare professional for a comprehensive evaluation to determine the specific causes of hypertension and develop an appropriate treatment plan. Managing hypertension involves a combination of lifestyle modifications, medication (if necessary), and regular monitoring to reduce the risk of complications and maintain optimal blood pressure levels.

CHAPTER 7

THE COMPLICATIONS THAT CAN ARISE FROM HYPERTENSION

Hypertension, or high blood pressure, if left uncontrolled or poorly managed, can lead to various complications that affect different organ systems in the body. Over time, the persistent elevation of blood pressure can damage blood vessels and strain the heart, increasing the risk of serious health problems.

Here are some of the common complications associated with hypertension:

Cardiovascular Disease:
Hypertension is a significant risk factor for the development of cardiovascular diseases. The constant high pressure in the arteries can damage the inner lining, leading to the formation of plaques, atherosclerosis (narrowing of the arteries), and decreased blood flow to the heart. This increases the risk

of heart attack, angina (chest pain), heart failure, and abnormal heart rhythms (arrhythmias).

Cardiovascular disease is one of the most significant and common complications that can arise from hypertension, also known as high blood pressure. Hypertension puts excessive strain on the heart and blood vessels, leading to long-term damage and increasing the risk of various cardiovascular conditions.

Here are key points about cardiovascular disease as a complication of hypertension:

1. Atherosclerosis: Hypertension contributes to the development and progression of atherosclerosis, a condition characterized by the buildup of fatty plaques inside the arteries. Elevated blood pressure damages the inner lining of the arteries, promoting the accumulation of cholesterol, fats, and other substances. Over time, these plaques can narrow the arteries, impeding blood flow to the heart and other organs.

2. Coronary Artery Disease (CAD): Hypertension is a major risk factor for coronary artery disease, a type of cardiovascular disease that affects the arteries supplying blood to the heart. The combination of hypertension and atherosclerosis can result in reduced blood flow to the heart muscle, leading to symptoms like angina (chest pain), shortness of breath, and in severe cases, heart attack.

3. Heart Attack (Myocardial Infarction): Hypertension can lead to the formation of blood clots within narrowed or damaged coronary arteries. If a blood clot completely blocks the blood flow to a part of the heart muscle, it can cause a heart attack. Heart attacks can cause permanent damage to the heart muscle and can be life-threatening.

4. Heart Failure: Persistent high blood pressure can strain the heart muscles, causing them to thicken and become less efficient at pumping blood. Over time, this can lead to heart failure, a condition where the heart is unable to pump blood effectively to meet the body's needs. Symptoms of heart failure include fatigue, shortness of breath, fluid retention, and swelling in the legs and ankles.

5. Arrhythmias: Hypertension can disrupt the normal electrical signaling in the heart, leading to abnormal heart rhythms or arrhythmias. This can manifest as a rapid heartbeat (tachycardia), an irregular heartbeat (atrial fibrillation), or other arrhythmias. Arrhythmias can increase the risk of stroke, heart failure, and other cardiovascular complications.

6. Hypertensive Heart Disease: Long-standing hypertension can result in structural changes in the heart, leading to hypertensive heart disease. This includes conditions such as left ventricular hypertrophy (enlargement and thickening of the heart's main pumping chamber) and diastolic dysfunction (impaired relaxation and filling of the heart chambers). These changes can impair heart function and increase the risk of heart failure.

7. Stroke: Hypertension is a major risk factor for stroke, a condition where the blood supply to the brain is interrupted. Persistent high blood pressure damages blood vessels in the brain, making them prone to blockages (ischemic stroke) or rupture (hemorrhagic stroke). Strokes can cause lasting neurological damage, disability, and in severe cases, death.

Managing hypertension effectively through lifestyle modifications (such as a healthy diet, regular exercise, stress reduction, and limiting alcohol and tobacco use) and, if necessary, medication prescribed by a healthcare professional, is crucial for preventing or minimizing the risk of cardiovascular complications. Regular monitoring of blood pressure, adherence to treatment plans, and regular check-ups are essential for early detection and management of hypertension-related cardiovascular disease. It is important to work closely with healthcare professionals to maintain optimal blood pressure control and reduce the risk of cardiovascular complications.

Stroke:

Uncontrolled hypertension can damage the blood
vessels in the brain, making them more susceptible to
blockages or rupture. This can result in a stroke, which
occurs when the blood supply to a part of the brain is
interrupted. Strokes can cause lasting brain damage,
paralysis, speech difficulties, and even be
life-threatening.

Stroke is a significant and potentially life-threatening
complication that can arise from hypertension,
commonly known as high blood pressure.
Hypertension places excessive strain on the blood
vessels, including those supplying the brain, increasing
the risk of stroke.

Here are key points about stroke as a complication of
hypertension:

1. Ischemic Stroke: The majority of strokes associated
with hypertension are ischemic strokes. In this type of
stroke, a blockage or clot forms in a blood vessel
supplying the brain, cutting off the blood supply to a

specific area. The elevated blood pressure damages the blood vessel walls, making them more prone to the formation of blood clots. The lack of blood flow and oxygen to the affected area of the brain leads to cell damage and potential long-term neurological consequences.

2. Hemorrhagic Stroke: Hypertension can also contribute to hemorrhagic strokes, although it is less common. In a hemorrhagic stroke, a weakened blood vessel ruptures, causing bleeding into the brain tissue. Chronic high blood pressure weakens the arterial walls, increasing the risk of rupture and bleeding. Hemorrhagic strokes can be particularly severe and life-threatening.

3. Risk Factors: Hypertension significantly increases the risk of stroke. Individuals with uncontrolled high blood pressure have a much higher likelihood of experiencing a stroke compared to those with normal blood pressure. Other risk factors for stroke, such as smoking, diabetes, high cholesterol, and obesity, often

coexist with hypertension, further compounding the
risk.

4. Consequences of Stroke: The consequences of
stroke can vary depending on the extent and location of
the brain damage. Common effects include paralysis or
weakness on one side of the body, difficulty speaking or
understanding speech (aphasia), vision problems,
coordination and balance issues, cognitive impairment,
and emotional changes. Stroke survivors may require
extensive rehabilitation and long-term care to regain
lost function and improve quality of life.

5. Prevention: Managing hypertension is crucial for
stroke prevention. Controlling blood pressure through
lifestyle modifications (such as adopting a healthy diet
low in sodium, regular exercise, weight management,
stress reduction, and limiting alcohol consumption)
and medications prescribed by healthcare professionals
can significantly reduce the risk of stroke. It is
important to follow the treatment plan provided by
healthcare professionals and maintain regular check-ups

to monitor blood pressure and adjust treatment as necessary.

6. Awareness and Prompt Treatment: Recognizing the signs and symptoms of stroke is essential for prompt medical intervention. The acronym FAST (Face drooping, Arm weakness, Speech difficulty, Time to call emergency services) is commonly used to identify potential stroke symptoms. If a stroke is suspected, it is crucial to seek immediate medical attention as early intervention can minimize brain damage and improve outcomes.

Hypertension management and stroke prevention go hand in hand. By effectively controlling blood pressure, adopting a healthy lifestyle, and working closely with healthcare professionals, individuals can significantly reduce the risk of stroke and its devastating consequences. Regular blood pressure monitoring, adherence to prescribed medications, and ongoing support from healthcare providers are vital components of stroke prevention in individuals with hypertension.

Kidney Disease:

The kidneys play a crucial role in regulating blood pressure. Chronic high blood pressure can damage the blood vessels in the kidneys, impairing their ability to filter waste and excess fluids from the body. This can lead to kidney disease, decreased kidney function, or even kidney failure, requiring dialysis or transplantation.

Kidney disease is a significant complication that can arise from hypertension, commonly known as high blood pressure. The kidneys play a crucial role in regulating blood pressure, and when hypertension is left uncontrolled or poorly managed, it can lead to damage to the blood vessels in the kidneys, impairing their function.

Here are key points about kidney disease as a complication of hypertension:

1. Hypertensive Nephropathy: Hypertensive nephropathy, also known as hypertensive kidney disease, refers to kidney damage caused by chronic high

95

blood pressure. The elevated pressure in the blood vessels of the kidneys can cause them to narrow and thicken, reducing blood flow and impairing the kidney's ability to effectively filter waste products and excess fluids from the body.

2. Chronic Kidney Disease (CKD): Long-standing hypertension can lead to the development and progression of chronic kidney disease. The damaged blood vessels in the kidneys can gradually impair their filtration function, resulting in the buildup of waste products and fluids in the body. CKD is characterized by a gradual loss of kidney function over time, which may ultimately progress to end-stage renal disease (ESRD), requiring dialysis or kidney transplantation.

3. Proteinuria: Hypertension can also cause damage to the filtering units of the kidneys, called nephrons. This can result in the leakage of proteins into the urine, a condition known as proteinuria. Persistent proteinuria is a sign of kidney damage and can further contribute to the progression of kidney disease.

4. Renal Artery Stenosis: Hypertension can lead to the narrowing of the renal arteries that supply blood to the kidneys, a condition called renal artery stenosis. The reduced blood flow to the kidneys triggers a cascade of events that can worsen hypertension and contribute to kidney damage.

5. Fluid and Electrolyte Imbalance: The kidneys play a crucial role in maintaining fluid balance and regulating electrolyte levels in the body. When kidney function is impaired due to hypertension-related damage, the kidneys may lose their ability to regulate these processes, leading to fluid retention, electrolyte imbalances, and potentially harmful complications.

6. Increased Cardiovascular Risk: Kidney disease, especially in the context of hypertension, increases the risk of developing cardiovascular complications. The damaged kidneys are less effective at filtering waste and excess fluids, leading to an increased burden on the cardiovascular system. Additionally, hypertension-related kidney disease is associated with a

higher risk of developing other cardiovascular
conditions, such as heart disease and stroke.

Management of hypertension is critical in preventing or
slowing the progression of kidney disease. Effective
blood pressure control through lifestyle modifications
(such as adopting a healthy diet low in sodium, regular
exercise, weight management, stress reduction, and
limiting alcohol consumption) and medications
prescribed by healthcare professionals can help protect
the kidneys and preserve their function. Regular
monitoring of blood pressure, kidney function, and
urine protein levels, as well as regular follow-up visits
with healthcare providers, are important for early
detection and management of hypertension-related
kidney disease.

It is important to note that individuals with pre-existing
kidney disease or those at increased risk should be
particularly vigilant in managing hypertension to
minimize the risk of further kidney damage. Healthcare
professionals play a crucial role in providing guidance,
monitoring kidney function, and adjusting treatment

plans to optimize blood pressure control and kidney health.

Eye Problems:

Hypertension can affect the blood vessels in the eyes, leading to damage to the retina (hypertensive retinopathy). It can cause vision problems, blurry vision, or even vision loss. In severe cases, it can result in retinal detachment or optic nerve damage, which may lead to permanent vision impairment.

Hypertension, commonly known as high blood pressure, can lead to various eye problems and complications. The persistent elevation of blood pressure can damage the blood vessels in the eyes, affecting their structure and function.

Here are key points about eye problems as complications of hypertension:

1. Hypertensive Retinopathy: Hypertensive retinopathy refers to changes in the blood vessels of the retina, the light-sensitive tissue at the back of the eye.

Elevated blood pressure can cause the blood vessels to narrow, leak, or become blocked, leading to retinal damage. This condition is characterized by the presence of changes such as narrowing of arteries, retinal hemorrhages (bleeding), cotton wool spots (small areas of nerve fiber layer infarction), and optic disc swelling. In severe cases, hypertensive retinopathy can result in vision loss or blindness.

2. Retinal Vein Occlusion: Hypertension increases the risk of retinal vein occlusion, a blockage in the veins that drain blood from the retina. The elevated pressure in the blood vessels can lead to the formation of blood clots, which can block the retinal veins, causing a sudden and significant decrease in vision. Retinal vein occlusion can result in permanent vision loss if not promptly diagnosed and treated.

3. Optic Neuropathy: Hypertension can contribute to optic neuropathy, which refers to damage to the optic nerve. The increased pressure in the blood vessels can disrupt blood flow to the optic nerve, leading to optic nerve damage and impaired vision. Optic neuropathy can manifest as vision loss, changes in color vision, or abnormalities in the visual field.

4. Vision Changes: Hypertension can cause vision changes that may include blurry vision, difficulty focusing, or fluctuations in vision. These changes are often temporary and can be related to fluctuations in blood pressure or changes in blood flow to the eyes.

5. Other Eye Conditions: Hypertension can also increase the risk or exacerbate other eye conditions, such as glaucoma (increased intraocular pressure damaging the optic nerve) and macular degeneration (deterioration of the central part of the retina). Individuals with hypertension may be more susceptible to the progression or complications of these conditions.

It is important for individuals with hypertension to prioritize regular eye examinations to monitor for any signs of eye problems or complications. Early detection and treatment can help prevent or minimize vision loss. Managing hypertension effectively through lifestyle modifications (such as a healthy diet, regular exercise,

stress reduction, and limiting alcohol and tobacco use)
and medications prescribed by healthcare professionals
is crucial for reducing the risk of eye-related
complications. Collaborating with healthcare
professionals and eye care specialists can help ensure
optimal blood pressure control and eye health,
minimizing the impact of hypertension on vision.

Peripheral Artery Disease:
Elevated blood pressure can contribute to the
development of peripheral artery disease, a condition
where the arteries in the legs and arms narrow or
become blocked. This can cause pain, numbness, and
difficulty walking or performing daily activities.

Peripheral artery disease (PAD) is a potential
complication that can arise from hypertension, also
known as high blood pressure. Hypertension can
contribute to the development and progression of
PAD, a condition characterized by the narrowing or
blockage of arteries that supply blood to the legs and
other peripheral areas of the body.

102

Here are key points about peripheral artery disease as a complication of hypertension:

1. Arterial Narrowing: Hypertension causes damage to the inner lining of blood vessels, promoting the accumulation of cholesterol, fats, and other substances, leading to atherosclerosis. Atherosclerosis can occur in arteries throughout the body, including the peripheral arteries. The narrowed arteries reduce blood flow to the muscles and tissues of the legs, resulting in symptoms such as leg pain, cramping, and weakness during physical activity, known as claudication.

2. Reduced Blood Supply: The narrowed or blocked arteries in PAD can limit the delivery of oxygen and nutrients to the affected limbs. This can lead to a variety of symptoms, including pain, numbness, and tingling in the legs or feet, especially during exercise or when at rest. In severe cases, inadequate blood supply can result in tissue damage, non-healing wounds, or even gangrene.

3. Increased Cardiovascular Risk: PAD is not only a localized condition but also an indicator of systemic atherosclerosis. Individuals with PAD are at an increased risk of other cardiovascular complications, including coronary artery disease, heart attack, and stroke. The presence of hypertension further amplifies this risk, as it contributes to the overall burden on the cardiovascular system.

4. Impaired Quality of Life: PAD can significantly impact an individual's quality of life. The limited blood flow to the legs and feet can cause pain and discomfort, making it challenging to walk or perform daily activities. The resulting mobility limitations can affect independence, social interactions, and overall well-being.

5. Ulcers and Wounds: In advanced cases of PAD, the compromised blood flow can lead to the development of ulcers or open sores on the legs or feet. These ulcers are often slow to heal and are prone to infection. Without proper management, they can lead to tissue damage and increase the risk of complications, such as amputation.

6. Prevention and Management: Managing hypertension is crucial for preventing or slowing the progression of PAD. Blood pressure control through lifestyle modifications (such as adopting a healthy diet low in sodium, regular exercise, weight management, stress reduction, and limiting alcohol consumption) and medications prescribed by healthcare professionals can help reduce the risk of PAD and its complications. Regular monitoring of blood pressure, early detection of PAD through diagnostic tests, and adherence to treatment plans are important in managing hypertension and preventing or managing PAD.

It is important for individuals with hypertension, particularly those with risk factors such as smoking, diabetes, or a family history of PAD, to be vigilant about their vascular health. Seeking medical attention for symptoms suggestive of PAD, such as leg pain or wounds that do not heal, is crucial for timely diagnosis and appropriate management. Healthcare professionals can provide guidance on lifestyle modifications, prescribe medications, and refer individuals to specialists when necessary to optimize blood pressure control and mitigate the impact of hypertension on peripheral artery disease.

Aneurysm:
Prolonged high blood pressure can weaken the walls of arteries, increasing the risk of an aneurysm. An aneurysm is a bulge or ballooning of a blood vessel that can rupture, leading to life-threatening internal bleeding.

Aneurysm is a potentially life-threatening complication that can arise from hypertension, commonly known as high blood pressure. Hypertension places excessive strain on the walls of blood vessels, weakening them and increasing the risk of developing an aneurysm.

Here are key points about aneurysms as a complication of hypertension:

1. Definition: An aneurysm is an abnormal bulging or ballooning of a blood vessel wall. It occurs when the weakened vessel wall cannot withstand the force of blood pressure, causing it to stretch and form a bulge. Aneurysms can develop in various arteries throughout the body, but they commonly occur in the aorta (the main artery that carries blood from the heart to the rest of the body) and the brain.

2. Aortic Aneurysms: Hypertension is a significant risk factor for the development and progression of aortic aneurysms. Chronic high blood pressure can weaken the walls of the aorta, making it more susceptible to the formation of an aneurysm. Aortic aneurysms can occur in the abdominal area (abdominal aortic aneurysm) or in the chest region (thoracic aortic aneurysm). If left untreated, aortic aneurysms can rupture, leading to life-threatening internal bleeding.

3. Cerebral Aneurysms: Hypertension also increases the risk of developing cerebral or brain aneurysms. These aneurysms occur in the blood vessels within the brain. The elevated blood pressure can put additional

stress on the weakened vessel walls, increasing the risk of
rupture and bleeding into the brain. Cerebral
aneurysms can cause a sudden and severe headache,
vision changes, neck pain, and neurological deficits if
they rupture.

4. Rupture and Hemorrhage: Aneurysms carry the
risk of rupture, which can result in severe bleeding. If
an aneurysm ruptures, it can cause life-threatening
internal bleeding within the affected organ or area. The
severity of the consequences depends on the location
and size of the aneurysm, as well as the extent of the
bleeding. Ruptured aneurysms require immediate
medical attention and can be a medical emergency.

5. Screening and Treatment: Screening for
aneurysms is not typically a routine part of
hypertension management. However, individuals with
hypertension who have additional risk factors, such as a
family history of aneurysms or other vascular diseases,
may be considered for screening tests, such as
ultrasound or imaging studies. Early detection of

aneurysms can facilitate timely intervention and
prevent rupture.

6. Blood Pressure Control: Effective management of
hypertension is crucial in reducing the risk of aneurysm
formation and rupture. Blood pressure control through
lifestyle modifications (such as adopting a healthy diet,
regular exercise, weight management, stress reduction,
and limiting alcohol consumption) and medications
prescribed by healthcare professionals can help reduce
the strain on blood vessel walls and decrease the risk of
aneurysm development or progression.

It is important for individuals with hypertension to
work closely with healthcare professionals to manage
their blood pressure effectively and reduce the risk of
complications such as aneurysms. Regular monitoring
of blood pressure, adherence to treatment plans, and
routine check-ups are vital in maintaining optimal
blood pressure control and minimizing the risk of
aneurysm formation or rupture. If an aneurysm is
detected, prompt evaluation by specialists and

appropriate treatment interventions can help prevent or
manage potential complications.

Metabolic Syndrome:
Hypertension is often associated with other metabolic
abnormalities, such as obesity, high cholesterol levels,
and insulin resistance. This cluster of conditions is
collectively known as metabolic syndrome, which
increases the risk of developing cardiovascular disease,
type 2 diabetes, and other health problems.

Metabolic syndrome is a cluster of conditions that can
arise as a complication of hypertension, also known as
high blood pressure. Metabolic syndrome refers to a
combination of several metabolic disorders, including
hypertension, obesity, dyslipidemia (abnormal lipid
levels), and insulin resistance. These conditions often
occur together and increase the risk of cardiovascular
disease and other health problems.

Here are key points about metabolic syndrome as a
complication of hypertension:

1. Hypertension as a Component: Hypertension is one of the key components of metabolic syndrome. Individuals with metabolic syndrome typically have elevated blood pressure, which contributes to the overall risk profile. The combination of hypertension with other metabolic abnormalities further amplifies the risk of developing cardiovascular complications.

2. Obesity: Obesity, particularly abdominal obesity, is another crucial component of metabolic syndrome. Excess body weight, especially around the waistline, is associated with increased blood pressure and insulin resistance. Obesity and hypertension often go hand in hand, and the presence of both conditions significantly raises the risk of heart disease, stroke, and type 2 diabetes.

3. Dyslipidemia: Metabolic syndrome often involves dyslipidemia, characterized by abnormal levels of lipids (cholesterol and triglycerides) in the blood. Individuals with metabolic syndrome commonly have elevated levels of low-density lipoprotein (LDL) cholesterol (known as "bad" cholesterol) and triglycerides, as well as decreased levels of high-density lipoprotein (HDL) cholesterol (known as "good" cholesterol). Dyslipidemia, combined with hypertension and obesity, contributes to the development of atherosclerosis and increases the risk of cardiovascular events.

4. Insulin Resistance: Insulin resistance is a hallmark of metabolic syndrome. It refers to a decreased ability of the body's cells to respond to insulin, a hormone responsible for regulating blood sugar levels. Insulin resistance leads to elevated blood glucose levels, which can contribute to the development of type 2 diabetes. Insulin resistance and hypertension are closely interconnected, as hypertension is commonly observed in individuals with insulin resistance.

5. Increased Cardiovascular Risk: Metabolic syndrome significantly raises the risk of developing cardiovascular disease. The combination of hypertension, obesity, dyslipidemia, and insulin resistance creates a pro-inflammatory and pro-thrombotic environment that promotes the formation of atherosclerotic plaques in blood vessels.

These plaques can narrow and harden the arteries, increasing the risk of heart attacks, strokes, and other cardiovascular events.

6. Comprehensive Management: Managing metabolic syndrome requires a comprehensive approach targeting multiple risk factors. Lifestyle modifications play a crucial role and include adopting a healthy diet, regular physical activity, weight management, and smoking cessation. Medications, such as antihypertensive drugs, lipid-lowering agents, and glucose-lowering medications, may be prescribed by healthcare professionals to manage individual components of metabolic syndrome.

Individuals with metabolic syndrome and hypertension should work closely with healthcare professionals to monitor and manage their condition effectively. Regular monitoring of blood pressure, lipid levels, blood glucose, and other relevant parameters is essential to assess the progress of treatment and adjust management strategies as needed. Lifestyle modifications, along with appropriate medications, can

113

help control blood pressure, improve lipid profiles, enhance insulin sensitivity, and reduce the risk of cardiovascular complications associated with metabolic syndrome and hypertension.

Cognitive Impairment:
Uncontrolled hypertension can have detrimental effects on brain health, contributing to cognitive decline, memory problems, and an increased risk of developing vascular dementia or Alzheimer's disease.

Cognitive impairment is a potential complication that can arise from hypertension, commonly known as high blood pressure. While hypertension primarily affects the cardiovascular system, it can also have detrimental effects on brain health and cognitive function.

Here are key points about cognitive impairment as a complication of hypertension:

1. Impact on Brain Health: Hypertension can damage blood vessels throughout the body, including those in the brain. The elevated pressure within the

114

blood vessels can cause small blood vessels in the brain to narrow, rupture, or become blocked. These vascular changes can disrupt blood flow to the brain, depriving it of oxygen and nutrients, and leading to brain damage over time. The brain areas affected by reduced blood flow are often associated with cognitive processes such as memory, attention, and executive functions.

2. Increased Risk of Cognitive Decline:

Long-standing or poorly controlled hypertension is associated with an increased risk of cognitive decline and the development of various cognitive impairments. Studies have shown that individuals with hypertension are more likely to experience problems with memory, attention, information processing speed, and executive functions compared to those with normal blood pressure. The cognitive decline may be gradual, occurring over a period of years, and can eventually progress to conditions such as mild cognitive impairment (MCI) or dementia.

3. Role of Hypertensive Encephalopathy: In severe cases, uncontrolled hypertension can lead to a condition

known as hypertensive encephalopathy. Hypertensive encephalopathy is characterized by a sudden and severe increase in blood pressure that can cause swelling and damage to the brain. This condition can manifest with symptoms such as headaches, confusion, seizures, and even coma. If left untreated, hypertensive encephalopathy can result in permanent brain damage and cognitive impairment.

4. Vascular Dementia: Hypertension is a significant risk factor for vascular dementia, a type of dementia caused by impaired blood flow to the brain. The damage to blood vessels in the brain can lead to the development of small vessel disease or multi-infarct dementia. Vascular dementia is characterized by a decline in cognitive abilities, including memory loss, difficulty with decision-making, and changes in behavior. It is important to note that hypertension can also coexist with other forms of dementia, such as Alzheimer's disease, further complicating cognitive impairment.

5. Prevention and Management: Effective management of hypertension is crucial for reducing the risk of cognitive impairment. Blood pressure control through lifestyle modifications (such as adopting a healthy diet low in sodium, regular exercise, weight management, stress reduction, and limiting alcohol consumption) and medications prescribed by healthcare professionals can help mitigate the impact of hypertension on brain health. Regular monitoring of blood pressure, routine check-ups, and adherence to treatment plans are essential in managing hypertension and potentially preventing or delaying cognitive decline.

It is important for individuals with hypertension to be aware of the potential impact on cognitive function and take proactive steps to manage their blood pressure effectively. Early detection and intervention are key in preventing or delaying cognitive impairment associated with hypertension. Seeking medical attention for symptoms suggestive of cognitive decline, such as memory problems or changes in thinking abilities, is crucial for evaluation and appropriate management.

117

Healthcare professionals can provide guidance on lifestyle modifications, prescribe medications, and offer support for maintaining optimal blood pressure control and preserving cognitive function.

It's important to note that the risk and severity of complications can vary among individuals, and not everyone with hypertension will experience all of these complications. However, by managing blood pressure effectively through lifestyle modifications (such as a healthy diet, regular exercise, stress reduction, and limiting alcohol and tobacco use) and, if necessary, medication prescribed by a healthcare professional, the risk of complications can be significantly reduced. Regular monitoring, adherence to treatment plans, and regular follow-up visits are essential to maintaining optimal blood pressure control and preventing or minimizing the impact of hypertension-related complications.

CHAPTER 8

LIFESTYLE CHANGES THAT CAN HELP MANAGE HYPERTENSION

Lifestyle changes play a crucial role in managing hypertension, also known as high blood pressure. By adopting healthy habits, individuals can effectively lower and control their blood pressure levels.

Here are some lifestyle changes that can help manage hypertension:

Healthy Diet:
Adopting a heart-healthy diet can have a significant impact on blood pressure. This includes consuming foods that are low in sodium (salt), saturated fats, and cholesterol. Instead, focus on incorporating fruits, vegetables, whole grains, lean proteins, and low-fat dairy products into your diet. The Dietary Approaches to Stop Hypertension (DASH) diet, which emphasizes fruits, vegetables, whole grains, lean proteins, and

119

low-fat dairy products, has been shown to be
particularly effective in reducing blood pressure.

Adopting a healthy diet is one of the most effective
lifestyle changes for managing hypertension, also
known as high blood pressure. A well-balanced and
nutrient-rich diet can significantly lower blood pressure
and reduce the risk of complications.

Here are key points about a healthy diet as a lifestyle
change for managing hypertension:

1. **DASH Diet:** The Dietary Approaches to Stop
Hypertension (DASH) diet is a well-researched eating
plan specifically designed to lower blood pressure. It
emphasizes fruits, vegetables, whole grains, lean
proteins, and low-fat dairy products while limiting
sodium, saturated fats, and cholesterol. The DASH diet
encourages portion control and promotes a
nutrient-rich and well-balanced approach to eating.

2. **Increase Fruits and Vegetables**: Incorporate a
variety of fruits and vegetables into your daily meals and

snacks. These foods are rich in essential vitamins, minerals, and dietary fiber, which contribute to overall cardiovascular health. Aim for at least five servings of fruits and vegetables per day, focusing on fresh, frozen, or canned options without added sugars or excessive sodium.

3. Whole Grains: Choose whole grains over refined grains whenever possible. Whole grains, such as whole wheat, oats, brown rice, and quinoa, provide more fiber and nutrients, which can help lower blood pressure. Incorporate whole grain bread, cereals, pasta, and rice into your diet instead of their refined counterparts.

4. Lean Proteins: Opt for lean sources of protein, such as skinless poultry, fish, legumes, and tofu. These protein sources are low in saturated fats and cholesterol, making them heart-healthy choices. Limit or avoid red meats, processed meats, and high-fat dairy products that are often high in saturated fats.

5. Low-Fat Dairy Products: Include low-fat or fat-free dairy products, such as milk, yogurt, and cheese,

121

as they are excellent sources of calcium and protein. These products provide the necessary nutrients without the added saturated fats and cholesterol found in full-fat dairy.

6. Limit Sodium Intake: Reduce your sodium (salt) intake by choosing low-sodium alternatives and minimizing the use of added salt when cooking or at the table. High sodium intake can contribute to elevated blood pressure. Read food labels, choose fresh or minimally processed foods, and avoid processed and packaged foods that tend to be high in sodium.

7. Potassium-Rich Foods: Include potassium-rich foods in your diet, as potassium helps regulate blood pressure. Good sources of potassium include bananas, oranges, spinach, sweet potatoes, tomatoes, and avocados. These foods can help counteract the effects of sodium and promote lower blood pressure levels.

8. Moderate Alcohol Consumption: If you consume alcohol, do so in moderation. Excessive alcohol intake can raise blood pressure. Moderate drinking is defined

122

as up to one drink per day for women and up to two drinks per day for men. However, it's important to note that for some individuals, it may be advisable to avoid alcohol altogether due to specific health conditions or medications.

9. Hydration: Stay well-hydrated by drinking an adequate amount of water each day. Proper hydration supports overall health and helps maintain normal blood pressure levels.

10. Mindful Eating: Practice mindful eating by paying attention to portion sizes, chewing food thoroughly, and savoring the flavors. This can help prevent overeating and promote a healthy relationship with food.

It is important to remember that dietary changes should be made in consultation with a healthcare professional or registered dietitian, particularly if you have underlying health conditions or unique dietary requirements. They can provide personalized guidance and support in developing a dietary plan tailored to your specific needs. By adopting a healthy diet, you can effectively manage hypertension, improve overall cardiovascular health, and reduce the risk of complications associated with high blood

Weight Management:

Maintaining a healthy weight is essential for managing hypertension. Losing excess weight, especially if you are overweight or obese, can significantly lower blood pressure. Aim for a gradual and sustainable weight loss by combining a balanced diet with regular physical activity.

Weight management is a crucial lifestyle change for managing hypertension, also known as high blood pressure. Maintaining a healthy weight is essential because excess body weight and obesity can significantly contribute to elevated blood pressure levels.

Here are key points about weight management as a lifestyle change for managing hypertension:

1. Relationship Between Weight and Blood Pressure: There is a strong association between excess body weight and hypertension. Carrying excess weight puts additional strain on the heart and blood vessels, leading to increased blood pressure. Losing weight can help reduce blood pressure levels and lower the risk of complications associated with hypertension.

2. Body Mass Index (BMI): Body Mass Index is a measurement that helps assess whether an individual has a healthy weight in relation to their height. Calculate your BMI to determine if you are within a healthy weight range. A BMI between 18.5 and 24.9 is considered normal, while a BMI of 25 or higher indicates overweight or obesity.

3. Gradual and Sustainable Weight Loss: Aim for a gradual and sustainable weight loss approach to avoid the pitfalls of fad diets or extreme measures. Losing weight at a rate of 1-2 pounds per week is generally considered safe and achievable. This can be accomplished through a combination of healthy eating, portion control, and regular physical activity.

4. Healthy Eating Habits: Adopting a balanced and nutritious diet is crucial for weight management. Focus on consuming a variety of fruits, vegetables, whole grains, lean proteins, and low-fat dairy products. Avoid or limit high-calorie and processed foods that are often low in nutritional value. Calorie intake should align with your specific energy needs based on age, sex, activity level, and weight goals.

5. Portion Control: Pay attention to portion sizes to avoid overeating. Be mindful of serving sizes recommended for different food groups and use measuring tools or portion-control aids if needed. Practice listening to your body's hunger and fullness cues to help regulate portion sizes effectively.

6. Regular Physical Activity: Engage in regular physical activity as part of your weight management plan. Exercise helps burn calories, improve cardiovascular health, and contribute to weight loss. Aim for at least 150 minutes of moderate-intensity aerobic exercise or 75 minutes of vigorous-intensity aerobic exercise per week. Additionally, incorporate strength training exercises at least twice a week to build muscle mass and boost metabolism.

7. Behavioral Changes: Adopting healthy behaviors is essential for long-term weight management. Be mindful of emotional eating triggers, stressors, or unhealthy habits that may contribute to weight gain. Develop strategies to cope with stress and emotions in ways that do not involve food, such as practicing relaxation techniques, engaging in hobbies, or seeking support from friends and family.

8. Support System: Seek support from healthcare professionals, registered dietitians, or support groups to help with weight management. They can provide guidance, personalized meal plans, and practical strategies to support your weight loss journey.

9. Regular Monitoring and Check-ups: Regularly monitor your weight and blood pressure levels to track your progress. Attend regular check-ups with your healthcare professional to assess overall health, adjust medications if necessary, and receive guidance on your weight management goals.

10. Sustainable Lifestyle Changes: Remember that weight management is a long-term commitment. Focus on adopting sustainable lifestyle changes rather than relying on short-term fixes. Healthy eating, regular physical activity, and weight management should become integral parts of your daily routine for optimal health and hypertension management.

It is important to consult with a healthcare professional before starting any weight loss program, especially if you have underlying health conditions or if you are taking medications. They can provide personalized guidance and support to ensure a safe and effective approach to weight management. By achieving and maintaining a healthy weight, you can significantly improve your blood pressure levels and reduce the risk of complications associated with hypertension.

Regular Physical Activity:

Engaging in regular physical activity can help lower
blood pressure and improve overall cardiovascular
health. Aim for at least 150 minutes of
moderate-intensity aerobic exercise or 75 minutes of
vigorous-intensity aerobic exercise each week, along
with strength training exercises at least twice a week.
Consult with your healthcare professional before
starting any exercise program, especially if you have
pre-existing health conditions.

Regular physical activity is an essential lifestyle change
for managing hypertension, also known as high blood
pressure. Engaging in regular exercise and staying
physically active has been shown to have numerous
benefits for blood pressure control and overall
cardiovascular health.

Here are key points about regular physical activity as a
lifestyle change for managing hypertension:

1. Blood Pressure Regulation: Regular physical
activity helps lower blood pressure by strengthening the

heart, improving blood flow, and promoting more efficient circulation. It can also contribute to the dilation of blood vessels, leading to lower resistance and reduced pressure on the arterial walls.

2. Aerobic Exercise: Aerobic exercises, such as brisk walking, jogging, cycling, swimming, and dancing, are particularly effective in lowering blood pressure. Aim for at least 150 minutes of moderate-intensity aerobic activity or 75 minutes of vigorous-intensity aerobic activity per week. You can break it down into smaller sessions throughout the week, such as 30 minutes on most days.

3. Strength Training: Incorporate strength training exercises at least two days a week. Strength training helps build muscle mass, increase metabolism, and improve overall physical strength. Include exercises that target major muscle groups, such as weightlifting, resistance band exercises, or bodyweight exercises like push-ups and squats.

4. Flexibility and Balance: In addition to aerobic and strength training, include flexibility and balance exercises in your routine. Stretching exercises can help improve flexibility, while balance exercises, such as yoga or tai chi, can enhance stability and coordination.

5. Start Slow and Progress Gradually: If you are new to exercise or have been inactive for a while, start with low-impact activities and gradually increase the intensity and duration over time. This allows your body to adapt and reduces the risk of injury. Consult with a healthcare professional or exercise specialist for personalized guidance, especially if you have underlying health conditions or concerns.

6. Enjoyable Activities: Choose physical activities that you enjoy and that suit your lifestyle. This increases the likelihood of sticking with the exercise regimen over the long term. Find activities that are convenient, fun, and align with your preferences, whether it's walking, dancing, swimming, cycling, or participating in team sports.

7. Consistency: Consistency is key in reaping the benefits of physical activity. Aim for regular exercise sessions throughout the week rather than sporadic bursts of activity. Create a schedule or routine that allows you to incorporate physical activity into your daily life. This helps make it a habit and ensures long-term adherence.

8. Monitor Intensity: Monitor the intensity of your physical activity to ensure it is appropriate for your fitness level. Aim for moderate-intensity exercise, where you can still talk but feel slightly breathless. If you have any concerns about the intensity or duration of exercise, consult with a healthcare professional or exercise specialist.

9. Be Active Throughout the Day: In addition to dedicated exercise sessions, find ways to stay active throughout the day. Take breaks from prolonged sitting, walk or bike for short errands, use stairs instead of elevators, or engage in household chores and gardening. These small lifestyle changes can add up and contribute to overall physical activity levels.

10. Safety Considerations: Prioritize safety during physical activity. Wear appropriate footwear and clothing, stay hydrated, and pay attention to your body's cues. If you experience any discomfort, pain, or unusual symptoms, stop exercising and consult with a healthcare professional.

Remember to consult with a healthcare professional before starting any exercise program, especially if you have underlying health conditions or if you are taking medications. They can provide personalized guidance and help design an exercise plan that is safe and effective for you. By incorporating regular physical activity into your lifestyle, you can effectively manage hypertension, improve cardiovascular health, and enhance overall well-being.

Sodium Reduction:
Excessive sodium intake can contribute to high blood pressure. Limiting sodium in your diet can help manage hypertension. Aim to consume no more than 2,300 milligrams (mg) of sodium per day, but ideally, try to

keep it under 1,500 mg per day. Read food labels, choose low-sodium alternatives, avoid processed foods, and limit the use of added salt when cooking or at the table.

Sodium reduction is an important lifestyle change for managing hypertension, also known as high blood pressure. Excess sodium intake can contribute to elevated blood pressure levels and increase the risk of cardiovascular complications. Adopting strategies to reduce sodium in your diet can help lower blood pressure and improve overall health.

Here are key points about sodium reduction as a lifestyle change for managing hypertension:

1. Understand Sodium's Role: Sodium is an essential mineral that plays a vital role in maintaining fluid balance and nerve function. However, excessive sodium intake can lead to water retention and increased blood pressure. The recommended daily sodium intake for most adults is 2,300 milligrams (mg) or less, with an

ideal target of 1,500 mg for individuals with
hypertension or other health conditions.

2. Read Food Labels: Start by reading food labels to
identify the sodium content in packaged and processed
foods. Pay attention to both the total sodium content
per serving and the recommended serving size. Choose
products labeled as "low sodium," "reduced sodium," or
"no added salt" whenever possible.

3. Cook from Scratch: Preparing meals at home using
fresh ingredients allows you to have greater control over
the amount of sodium in your diet. Focus on using
fresh fruits, vegetables, lean proteins, and whole grains.
Limit the use of processed foods, as they tend to be
higher in sodium.

4. Limit Processed and Packaged Foods: Processed
and packaged foods, such as canned soups, sauces,
condiments, deli meats, and snacks, are often high in
sodium. Opt for fresh or frozen alternatives whenever
possible, as they generally have lower sodium content. If
you do choose packaged foods, look for lower sodium

options or rinse canned foods, like beans or vegetables, before consuming to reduce sodium levels.

5. Be Mindful of Hidden Sodium: Sodium can be found in unexpected places, including bread, cheese, salad dressings, and even breakfast cereals. Be mindful of these hidden sources of sodium and choose lower sodium options or make your own dressings and sauces using herbs, spices, and other flavorings.

6. Flavor with Herbs and Spices: Enhance the taste of your meals by using herbs, spices, and other flavorful ingredients instead of relying on salt. Experiment with garlic, onion, lemon juice, vinegar, black pepper, oregano, basil, and other herbs and spices to add depth and flavor to your dishes.

7. Limit Salt in Cooking and at the Table: Reduce the amount of salt you add during cooking and at the table. Gradually decrease the amount of salt used in recipes and experiment with other seasonings to enhance the taste of your meals. Over time, your taste buds will adjust to lower sodium levels.

8. Choose Fresh and Whole Foods: Fresh fruits, vegetables, and whole grains are naturally low in sodium and rich in other beneficial nutrients. Include a variety of these foods in your diet to support overall health and blood pressure management.

9. Be Cautious with Condiments and Sauces: Condiments and sauces, such as soy sauce, ketchup, mustard, and barbecue sauce, can be high in sodium. Opt for low-sodium versions or use them sparingly. Consider alternatives like fresh salsa, homemade dressings, or herbs and spices to add flavor to your dishes.

10. Seek Support and Guidance: If you find it challenging to reduce sodium in your diet or need assistance in creating a low-sodium meal plan, consider consulting with a registered dietitian. They can provide personalized guidance and practical tips to help you manage your sodium intake effectively.

Remember that reducing sodium intake should be part of an overall healthy eating plan. It is important to focus on a balanced diet that includes other nutrient-rich foods and lifestyle factors, such as regular physical activity and weight management, for optimal

Limit Alcohol Consumption:
Drinking excessive amounts of alcohol can raise blood pressure. If you choose to drink alcohol, do so in moderation. Men should limit their alcohol intake to a maximum of two standard drinks per day, and women should limit their intake to one standard drink per day. It is important to note that excessive alcohol consumption can have detrimental effects on overall health, so it is best to consult with your healthcare professional regarding alcohol consumption and its impact on your specific health condition.

Limiting alcohol consumption is an important lifestyle change for managing hypertension, also known as high blood pressure. Excessive alcohol intake can contribute to elevated blood pressure levels and increase the risk of cardiovascular complications. Adopting strategies to

reduce alcohol consumption can help lower blood
pressure and improve overall health.

Here are key points about limiting alcohol
consumption as a lifestyle change for managing
hypertension:

1. Understand the Relationship: Alcohol
consumption, particularly heavy or excessive drinking,
can lead to high blood pressure. Alcohol affects the
sympathetic nervous system, which controls blood
vessel constriction and heart rate. It can also damage the
arteries and lead to inflammation, contributing to
hypertension.

2. Know the Recommended Limits: The
recommended limits for alcohol consumption vary by
country and gender. In general, it is advised to limit
alcohol intake to moderate levels. For men, this means
up to two standard drinks per day, while for women, it
is recommended to have up to one standard drink per
day. It's important to note that some individuals, such
as those with certain medical conditions or taking

specific medications, may need to avoid alcohol
altogether.

3. Measure Serving Sizes: Be aware of what
constitutes a standard drink. A standard drink typically
contains about 14 grams of pure alcohol, which is
equivalent to 1.5 ounces (44 milliliters) of distilled
spirits, 5 ounces (148 milliliters) of wine, or 12 ounces
(355 milliliters) of beer. It's easy to exceed the
recommended limits if you're not mindful of the actual
serving sizes.

4. Be Mindful of Mixed Drinks and Cocktails:
Mixed drinks and cocktails can contain high amounts
of alcohol and added sugars, which can contribute to
weight gain and elevated blood pressure. Limit your
consumption of these types of beverages or opt for
lower-alcohol alternatives, such as spritzers or light
beers.

5. Pace Yourself and Take Breaks: If you choose to
drink, pace yourself and take breaks between alcoholic
beverages. Avoid binge drinking, which is defined as

consuming a large amount of alcohol within a short period. Instead, savor your drink and alternate with non-alcoholic beverages, such as water or sparkling water, to stay hydrated.

6. Avoid Excessive Drinking: Excessive or heavy drinking significantly increases the risk of developing hypertension and other health problems. It is defined as consuming more than the recommended limits on a regular basis. If you have hypertension or are at risk, it is advisable to limit or avoid alcohol altogether.

7. Seek Support: If you find it challenging to limit your alcohol consumption, seek support from healthcare professionals, support groups, or counseling services. They can provide guidance, resources, and strategies to help you make positive changes and manage your alcohol intake effectively.

8. Be Aware of Triggers and Alternatives: Identify triggers or situations that may lead to excessive alcohol consumption and develop strategies to manage them. Find alternative activities or beverages to replace

alcohol, such as engaging in hobbies, exercise, or
enjoying alcohol-free mocktails.

9. Educate Yourself on the Risks: Educate yourself
about the risks associated with excessive alcohol
consumption, especially when combined with
hypertension. Understand how alcohol affects your
body and the potential consequences it may have on
your blood pressure and overall health.

10. Regularly Monitor Blood Pressure: Regularly
monitor your blood pressure levels to track the impact
of alcohol reduction on your hypertension
management. Consult with a healthcare professional to
determine the appropriate frequency of blood pressure
checks and discuss any changes or concerns.

Remember that lifestyle changes, including limiting
alcohol consumption, work best when combined with
other healthy habits such as a balanced diet, regular
physical activity, weight management, and stress
reduction. If you have concerns or questions about
alcohol consumption and its impact on your blood

pressure, consult with a healthcare professional for personalized guidance and support.

Quit Smoking:
Smoking and using tobacco products can raise blood pressure and damage blood vessels. Quitting smoking is a critical step in managing hypertension and improving overall cardiovascular health. Seek support from healthcare professionals, join smoking cessation programs, or explore nicotine replacement therapies to aid in the quitting process.

Quitting smoking is a crucial lifestyle change for managing hypertension, also known as high blood pressure. Smoking and hypertension have a synergistic effect on cardiovascular health, increasing the risk of heart disease, stroke, and other complications. Quitting smoking not only improves blood pressure control but also provides a range of overall health benefits.

Here are key points about quitting smoking as a lifestyle change for managing hypertension:

143

1. Understand the Connection: Smoking tobacco causes a temporary increase in blood pressure and damages blood vessels, leading to chronic hypertension over time. The chemicals in tobacco smoke can also promote inflammation and the formation of plaque in the arteries, further contributing to cardiovascular disease.

2. Seek Professional Help: Quitting smoking can be challenging due to nicotine addiction and behavioral patterns. Seek professional help to increase your chances of success. Consult with healthcare professionals, such as doctors, counselors, or smoking cessation specialists, who can provide guidance, support, and resources to assist you in the quitting process.

3. Develop a Quit Plan: Create a personalized quit plan that includes setting a quit date, identifying triggers, and outlining coping strategies. Determine the approach that suits you best, whether it's quitting abruptly or gradually reducing your smoking over time. Consider utilizing nicotine replacement therapies, medications, or behavioral therapies as recommended by healthcare professionals.

4. Support Systems: Inform your friends, family, and colleagues about your decision to quit smoking. Their support and encouragement can make a significant difference. Consider joining smoking cessation support groups or online communities to connect with individuals who are going through a similar journey.

5. Identify and Avoid Triggers: Identify situations or factors that typically trigger the urge to smoke and develop strategies to avoid or manage them. For example, if certain social settings or routines make you crave a cigarette, find alternative activities to engage in or modify your routine to break the association.

6. Replace Smoking with Healthy Habits: Replace smoking with healthier habits to cope with cravings and reduce stress. Engage in physical activity, practice relaxation techniques like deep breathing or meditation, or find other enjoyable activities that can distract you from the urge to smoke.

7. Be Prepared for Withdrawal Symptoms:

Nicotine withdrawal symptoms may occur when you quit smoking. These symptoms can include irritability, anxiety, restlessness, difficulty concentrating, and cravings. Understand that these symptoms are temporary and will subside over time. Implement healthy coping strategies, such as exercise, deep breathing, or engaging in hobbies, to manage withdrawal symptoms.

8. Focus on Health Benefits: Remind yourself of the numerous health benefits of quitting smoking. Within minutes of quitting, blood pressure starts to decrease, and within weeks, lung function improves. Over time, the risk of heart disease, stroke, and other smoking-related health conditions decreases significantly.

9. Celebrate Milestones: Celebrate milestones along your journey to becoming smoke-free. Acknowledge and reward yourself for every day, week, or month that you remain smoke-free. Treat yourself to something you

enjoy or invest in a reward that supports your overall
health and well-being.

10. Stay Committed: Quitting smoking is a process
that requires commitment, perseverance, and
determination. It's normal to experience setbacks or
relapses, but it's important to learn from them and keep
moving forward. Don't get discouraged by temporary
setbacks and remind yourself of the benefits of a
smoke-free life.

Remember, quitting smoking is one of the most
significant steps you can take to improve your health
and manage hypertension. It's never too late to quit,
and the sooner you quit, the greater the benefits. Seek
support, stay motivated, and celebrate your progress
along the way. With determination and support, you
can successfully quit smoking and significantly reduce
the risks associated with hypertension and other
smoking-related diseases.

Stress Management:

Chronic stress can contribute to high blood pressure. Finding healthy ways to manage stress, such as practicing relaxation techniques (e.g., deep breathing exercises, meditation, yoga), engaging in hobbies, spending time with loved ones, and participating in activities that bring joy and relaxation, can help reduce blood pressure and promote overall well-being.

Stress management is a vital lifestyle change for managing hypertension, also known as high blood pressure. Chronic stress can contribute to elevated blood pressure levels and negatively impact cardiovascular health. Implementing effective stress management techniques can help reduce stress, promote relaxation, and improve overall well-being.

Here are key points about stress management as a lifestyle change for managing hypertension:

1. Recognize Stress Triggers: Identify the factors that contribute to stress in your life. These may include work pressure, relationship issues, financial concerns, or other personal challenges. Understanding your stress triggers is the first step in effectively managing stress.

2. Practice Relaxation Techniques: Engage in relaxation techniques to counteract the physiological and psychological effects of stress. Deep breathing exercises, meditation, progressive muscle relaxation, and guided imagery are all effective relaxation techniques that can help reduce stress levels and promote a sense of calm.

3. Physical Activity and Exercise: Regular physical activity and exercise have been shown to reduce stress and lower blood pressure. Engaging in activities like walking, jogging, swimming, cycling, or yoga can help alleviate stress and promote overall cardiovascular health. Aim for at least 150 minutes of moderate-intensity aerobic activity or 75 minutes of vigorous-intensity aerobic activity each week.

4. Time Management and Prioritization: Effective time management and prioritization can help reduce stress by creating a sense of control and organization in your life. Prioritize tasks, set realistic goals, and break larger tasks into smaller, manageable steps. Avoid overcommitting and learn to delegate or say no when necessary.

5. Establish Healthy Boundaries: Setting boundaries is essential for managing stress. Learn to assertively communicate your needs and limits, both in personal and professional relationships. Avoid taking on excessive responsibilities or allowing others to infringe upon your personal time and well-being.

6. Social Support: Surround yourself with a supportive network of family, friends, or support groups. Share your concerns, seek advice, and lean on others for emotional support. Connecting with others who are experiencing similar challenges can provide validation and a sense of community.

7. Healthy Coping Mechanisms: Adopt healthy coping mechanisms to manage stress rather than relying on unhealthy habits like smoking, excessive alcohol consumption, or overeating. Engage in activities you enjoy, such as hobbies, reading, listening to music, or spending time in nature.

8. Adequate Sleep: Prioritize quality sleep as it plays a crucial role in stress management and overall well-being. Establish a regular sleep routine, create a comfortable sleep environment, and practice good sleep hygiene habits. Aim for 7-8 hours of quality sleep each night.

9. Mindfulness and Mind-Body Techniques: Cultivate mindfulness by focusing on the present moment and practicing non-judgmental awareness. Mind-body techniques such as yoga, tai chi, and qigong combine physical movement, breath control, and meditation, promoting relaxation and stress reduction.

10. Seek Professional Help: If you're experiencing persistent or overwhelming stress, consider seeking professional help. Mental health professionals, such as therapists or counselors, can provide guidance and support in developing effective stress management strategies tailored to your specific needs.

It's important to note that stress management is a continuous practice, and what works for one person may not work for another. Explore different techniques, be patient with yourself, and find what resonates with you. By actively managing stress, you can significantly reduce its impact on your blood pressure and overall health, improving your ability to manage hypertension effectively.

Regular Monitoring and Healthcare Visits:
Regular monitoring of blood pressure is essential to track your progress and adjust lifestyle modifications or medication as needed. Additionally, maintaining regular visits with your healthcare professional ensures proper management and monitoring of hypertension.

Regular monitoring and healthcare visits are essential lifestyle changes for effectively managing hypertension, also known as high blood pressure. Monitoring your blood pressure levels and maintaining regular contact with healthcare professionals are crucial steps in controlling hypertension and preventing associated complications.

Here are key points about regular monitoring and
healthcare visits as lifestyle changes for managing
hypertension:

1. Blood Pressure Monitoring: Regularly monitor
your blood pressure levels at home using a reliable
blood pressure monitor. Keep a record of your readings
and share them with your healthcare provider during
your visits. This helps you track changes in your blood
pressure over time and provides valuable information
for adjusting treatment plans if necessary.

2. Know Your Target Blood Pressure Range:
Understand your target blood pressure range as
determined by your healthcare provider. In general, the
target for most individuals with hypertension is a
systolic blood pressure (the top number) below 130
mmHg and a diastolic blood pressure (the bottom
number) below 80 mmHg. However, your target may
vary depending on your overall health and any other
underlying medical conditions you may have.

3. Regular Healthcare Visits: Schedule regular appointments with your healthcare provider to monitor and manage your hypertension. These visits allow your doctor to assess your blood pressure readings, review your overall health, adjust medications if necessary, and provide guidance on lifestyle modifications.

4. Medication Management: If you are prescribed medications to control your blood pressure, it is crucial to take them as prescribed by your healthcare provider. Regular healthcare visits allow your doctor to monitor the effectiveness of your medications, make adjustments if needed, and address any concerns or side effects you may be experiencing.

5. Health Assessments and Screenings: Regular healthcare visits provide an opportunity for comprehensive health assessments and screenings. Your healthcare provider may conduct tests to assess your cholesterol levels, blood sugar levels, kidney function, and other parameters related to your cardiovascular health. These assessments help identify and manage any underlying conditions that may contribute to hypertension or its complications.

6. Lifestyle Counseling: Healthcare visits offer an opportunity for lifestyle counseling. Your healthcare provider can provide guidance and support in making necessary lifestyle changes, such as adopting a healthy diet, engaging in regular physical activity, quitting smoking, managing stress, and reducing alcohol consumption. They can also address any specific concerns or challenges you may have regarding your lifestyle modifications.

7. Education and Empowerment: Regular healthcare visits allow you to stay informed about hypertension, its management, and potential complications. Your healthcare provider can educate you about the condition, answer your questions, and empower you with knowledge to actively participate in your own care.

8. Individualized Treatment Plans: Every individual's hypertension management plan may differ based on their unique health profile. Regular healthcare visits ensure that your treatment plan is regularly reviewed and adjusted to meet your specific needs and goals. It allows your healthcare provider to tailor your treatment approach and provide personalized recommendations.

9. Early Detection and Prevention: Regular monitoring and healthcare visits help in the early detection of any changes or complications related to hypertension. By detecting and addressing potential issues promptly, you can prevent further progression of the condition and reduce the risk of associated complications.

10. Collaboration and Support: Regular healthcare visits foster a collaborative relationship between you and your healthcare provider. It provides an opportunity for open communication, sharing of concerns, and receiving ongoing support in managing your hypertension effectively.

Remember, managing hypertension requires a proactive and comprehensive approach. Regular monitoring of your blood pressure, maintaining contact with healthcare professionals, and actively engaging in your own care can significantly improve your ability to control blood pressure levels, reduce complications, and lead a healthier life.

Remember, lifestyle changes should be implemented in consultation with your healthcare professional, who can provide personalized recommendations based on your specific health condition and individual needs. By incorporating these lifestyle changes into your daily routine, you can take an active role in managing your hypertension and promoting overall cardiovascular health.

CHAPTER 9

MEDICAL TREATMENTS FOR HYPERTENSION

Medical treatments for hypertension, also known as high blood pressure, aim to reduce and control blood pressure levels to prevent complications and promote overall cardiovascular health. While lifestyle modifications play a crucial role in managing hypertension, medications are often prescribed when lifestyle changes alone are insufficient. It's important to note that medical treatments should be determined and prescribed by healthcare professionals based on an individual's specific health profile. Here are some common medical treatments for hypertension:

Medications

1. Angiotensin-Converting Enzyme (ACE) Inhibitors:

ACE inhibitors block the production of angiotensin II, a hormone that constricts blood vessels, thereby reducing blood pressure. These medications also help in reducing the workload on the heart. Examples include lisinopril, enalapril, and ramipril.

2. Angiotensin II Receptor Blockers (ARBs):

ARBs work by blocking the action of angiotensin II, preventing it from narrowing blood vessels. This helps lower blood pressure. Some commonly prescribed ARBs include losartan, valsartan, and candesartan.

3. Diuretics:

Diuretics, often referred to as water pills, help the kidneys eliminate excess sodium and water from the body, reducing the volume of blood and lowering blood pressure. They are available in different types, including thiazide diuretics (such as hydrochlorothiazide), loop diuretics (such as furosemide), and potassium-sparing diuretics (such as spironolactone).

4. Calcium Channel Blockers (CCBs):

CCBs relax and widen the blood vessels, allowing for smoother blood flow and reducing blood pressure.

They also have a relaxing effect on the heart. Examples include amlodipine, diltiazem, and verapamil.

5. Beta-Blockers:

Beta-blockers work by blocking the effects of adrenaline, a hormone that increases heart rate and blood pressure. They slow down the heart rate and reduce the force of contraction, lowering blood pressure. Some commonly prescribed beta-blockers are metoprolol, propranolol, and atenolol.

6. Renin Inhibitors:

Renin inhibitors, such as aliskiren, work by inhibiting the production of renin, an enzyme involved in the production of angiotensin II. By reducing the levels of angiotensin II, blood vessels can relax and blood pressure can be lowered.

7. Alpha-Blockers:

Alpha-blockers relax the muscles in the walls of blood vessels, allowing them to widen and reducing resistance to blood flow. This helps lower blood pressure. Examples include doxazosin, prazosin, and terazosin.

8. Combination Medications:

In some cases, a single medication may not be sufficient to control blood pressure. Combination medications that contain two or more blood pressure-lowering agents in a single pill may be prescribed. This approach helps simplify the medication regimen and improve adherence.

9. Other Medications:

In certain situations, additional medications may be prescribed to manage specific underlying conditions or risk factors contributing to hypertension. For example, medications to lower cholesterol (statins), control blood sugar (antidiabetic medications), or prevent blood clot formation (anticoagulants) may be prescribed.

Surgical Procedures:

1. Renal Denervation:

Renal denervation is a minimally invasive procedure that involves disrupting the nerves in the kidneys responsible for regulating blood pressure. This

procedure is typically reserved for individuals with
resistant hypertension who do not respond well to
medications.

2. Bariatric Surgery:

Bariatric surgery may be recommended for individuals
with severe obesity and hypertension. Weight loss
resulting from the surgery can lead to significant
improvements in blood pressure control.

3. Other Surgical Interventions:

In rare cases, surgical procedures may be performed to
address specific underlying conditions contributing to
hypertension. For example, surgery to remove a tumor
causing excessive hormone production or to repair
narrowed blood vessels may be considered.

Regular monitoring of blood pressure and follow-up
visits with healthcare providers are essential to evaluate
the effectiveness of the chosen treatment approach and
make any necessary adjustments. Additionally, lifestyle
modifications, such as adopting a healthy diet, engaging
in regular physical activity, managing stress, and

limiting alcohol consumption, are often recommended
alongside medical treatments to optimize blood
pressure control and overall cardiovascular health.

It's important to follow the prescribed dosage and
frequency of medications as advised by healthcare
professionals. Regular monitoring of blood pressure
and periodic follow-up visits with healthcare providers
are essential to assess the effectiveness of the prescribed
medications and make any necessary adjustments.

It's worth noting that the choice of medication may
vary depending on individual factors, such as age,
overall health, presence of other medical conditions,
and potential side effects. Healthcare professionals
consider these factors when tailoring the treatment plan
to best suit each

CHAPTER 10

ALTERNATIVE THERAPIES FOR HYPERTENSION

Alternative therapies, also known as complementary and integrative approaches, are non-conventional treatment options that can be used alongside or in combination with medical treatments for hypertension. While they should not replace medical advice or prescribed medications, some individuals may find these therapies helpful in managing their blood pressure. It is important to consult with a healthcare professional before starting any alternative therapy.

Here are some alternative therapies that have been explored for hypertension:

Relaxation Techniques:
Techniques such as deep breathing exercises, progressive muscle relaxation, meditation, and guided imagery can help reduce stress and promote relaxation. Stress reduction techniques may have a positive impact on

blood pressure by reducing sympathetic nervous system activity and promoting vasodilation.

Biofeedback:

Biofeedback involves using electronic devices to monitor and provide feedback on certain physiological processes, such as heart rate, blood pressure, and muscle tension. It helps individuals become more aware of their body's response to stress and learn techniques to control these responses, potentially leading to better blood pressure control.

Acupuncture:

Acupuncture is an ancient Chinese practice that involves inserting thin needles into specific points on the body. Some studies suggest that acupuncture may help lower blood pressure by promoting relaxation, improving blood flow, and reducing sympathetic nervous system activity. However, more research is needed to establish its effectiveness for hypertension.

Herbal Supplements:

Certain herbal supplements, such as garlic extract, hawthorn extract, and fish oil, have been studied for their potential benefits in managing blood pressure. However, the evidence is limited, and it's important to consult with a healthcare professional before using any herbal supplements as they may interact with prescribed medications.

Dietary Supplements:

Some dietary supplements, including coenzyme Q10 (CoQ10), omega-3 fatty acids, and magnesium, have been studied for their potential role in blood pressure management. However, more research is needed to determine their effectiveness and safety for hypertension. It is important to discuss the use of dietary supplements with a healthcare provider before incorporating them into a treatment plan.

Mind-Body Interventions:

Practices like yoga, tai chi, and qigong combine physical movement, breathing techniques, and mindfulness. These mind-body interventions may help

166

reduce stress, improve cardiovascular health, and promote overall well-being. They may be beneficial as part of a comprehensive approach to managing hypertension.

Dietary Approaches:

Certain dietary approaches, such as the Dietary Approaches to Stop Hypertension (DASH) diet, emphasize consuming a diet rich in fruits, vegetables, whole grains, lean proteins, and low-fat dairy products while limiting sodium, saturated fats, and processed foods. The DASH diet has been shown to help lower blood pressure and is often recommended alongside medical treatments.

It's important to note that the effectiveness of alternative therapies for hypertension can vary among individuals, and their impact on blood pressure may be modest compared to medical treatments. Moreover, some alternative therapies may have potential risks and interactions with prescribed medications. Therefore, it is crucial to consult with a healthcare professional before incorporating any alternative therapies into your

hypertension management plan. They can provide
guidance, monitor your progress, and ensure the
therapies are safe and appropriate for your specific
health condition.

CHAPTER 11

STRATEGIES FOR MONITORING AND MANAGING HYPERTENSION

Monitoring and managing hypertension requires a proactive approach that includes regular check-ups, self-monitoring, and goal-setting.

Here are some strategies to help effectively monitor and manage hypertension:

Regular Check-ups:
Schedule regular check-ups with your healthcare provider to monitor your blood pressure and overall health. During these visits, your healthcare provider can assess your blood pressure readings, review your medical history, discuss any symptoms or concerns, and adjust your treatment plan if necessary. Regular check-ups help ensure that your hypertension is being properly managed and allow for early detection of any potential complications.

Self-Monitoring:

Self-monitoring of blood pressure at home is an important tool in managing hypertension. Your healthcare provider can guide you on how to use a home blood pressure monitor correctly. Regularly measure your blood pressure at home and keep a record of the readings. This information will help you and your healthcare provider track your blood pressure trends and make informed decisions about your treatment plan.

Goal-Setting:

Work with your healthcare provider to set realistic goals for blood pressure control. These goals may be based on recommended blood pressure targets for your specific situation. Aim to achieve and maintain a blood pressure reading below the recommended target. By setting clear goals, you can track your progress and stay motivated to make the necessary lifestyle changes and adhere to your treatment plan.

Medication Adherence:

If prescribed medication to manage your hypertension, take it as directed by your healthcare provider. Adherence to your medication regimen is crucial for maintaining optimal blood pressure control. If you have concerns or experience side effects, discuss them with your healthcare provider, who may be able to adjust your medication or provide alternative options.

Healthy Lifestyle Modifications:

Make lifestyle changes that promote better blood pressure control.

These include:

1. Healthy Diet: Adopt a balanced diet rich in fruits, vegetables, whole grains, lean proteins, and low-fat dairy products. Reduce sodium (salt) intake and limit processed and high-sodium foods.

2. Regular Exercise: Engage in regular physical activity, such as brisk walking, swimming, cycling, or other forms of aerobic exercise. Aim for at least 150 minutes of moderate-intensity exercise or 75 minutes of vigorous-intensity exercise per week, or as recommended by your healthcare provider.

3. Weight Management: If overweight or obese, strive to achieve and maintain a healthy weight through a combination of healthy eating and regular physical activity. Even modest weight loss can have a positive impact on blood pressure.

4. Sodium Reduction: Limit your sodium intake by avoiding or minimizing processed and packaged foods, which often contain high levels of sodium. Read food labels and choose low-sodium alternatives whenever possible.

5. Stress Management: Practice stress-reducing techniques such as deep breathing exercises, meditation, yoga, or engaging in hobbies and activities that promote relaxation and well-being.

Educate Yourself:

Learn about hypertension, its management, and potential complications. Understand the importance of lifestyle modifications and medication adherence in controlling blood pressure. Stay informed about the latest guidelines and recommendations related to hypertension management.

Support Network:

Seek support from family, friends, or support groups. Sharing experiences and learning from others who are managing hypertension can provide valuable encouragement, motivation, and accountability.

Remember to consult your healthcare provider before making any significant changes to your treatment plan or lifestyle. They can provide personalized guidance based on your specific situation and help you develop a comprehensive strategy for monitoring and managing your hypertension effectively.

CHAPTER 12

HOW TO PREVENT HYPERTENSION

Preventing hypertension involves adopting a healthy lifestyle and minimizing risk factors. By making positive changes to your daily habits and overall well-being, you can significantly reduce the risk of developing hypertension.

Here are some tips for preventing hypertension:

Maintain a Healthy Weight:
 Aim for a body mass index (BMI) within the normal range. Losing excess weight, if necessary, through a combination of healthy eating and regular physical activity can help reduce the risk of hypertension.

Follow a Healthy Diet:
Emphasize a balanced diet that includes fruits, vegetables, whole grains, lean proteins, and low-fat dairy products. Limit the consumption of saturated fats, trans fats, cholesterol, sodium (salt), and added

sugars. The Dietary Approaches to Stop Hypertension (DASH) diet is specifically designed to help lower blood pressure and is recommended for individuals at risk of or already diagnosed with hypertension.

Reduce Sodium Intake:

Limit the amount of sodium in your diet. Avoid adding salt to your meals and choose low-sodium alternatives when shopping for packaged and processed foods. Read food labels carefully to make informed choices.

Exercise Regularly:

Engage in regular physical activity for at least 150 minutes of moderate-intensity aerobic exercise or 75 minutes of vigorous-intensity exercise per week. Incorporate activities that you enjoy, such as walking, jogging, swimming, cycling, or dancing, into your routine. Consult with your healthcare provider before starting any exercise program.

Limit Alcohol Consumption:

If you drink alcohol, do so in moderation. Limit intake to up to one drink per day for women and up to two drinks per day for men. Excessive alcohol consumption can raise blood pressure and contribute to other health problems.

Quit Smoking:

Smoking damages blood vessels and raises blood pressure. If you smoke, seek assistance from healthcare professionals to quit smoking. Quitting smoking can greatly improve your overall health and reduce the risk of hypertension and other cardiovascular diseases.

Manage Stress:

Chronic stress can contribute to the development of hypertension. Practice stress-management techniques such as deep breathing exercises, meditation, yoga, or engaging in activities that help you relax and unwind. Find healthy outlets to manage stress, such as hobbies, spending time with loved ones, or pursuing activities you enjoy.

Get Regular Check-Ups:

Schedule regular check-ups with your healthcare provider. Routine screenings and monitoring of blood pressure can help detect any changes early and allow for timely interventions or lifestyle modifications.

Know Your Family History:
Be aware of your family's medical history, as hypertension can have a genetic component. Inform your healthcare provider about any family history of hypertension or other cardiovascular diseases.

Educate Yourself:
Learn about the risk factors, symptoms, and complications associated with hypertension. Stay informed about current guidelines and recommendations for blood pressure management. This knowledge will empower you to make informed decisions about your health and take necessary steps to prevent hypertension.

Remember, prevention is key to maintaining optimal health. By adopting a healthy lifestyle, managing risk factors, and seeking regular medical care, you can significantly reduce the likelihood of developing hypertension and promote overall well-being. If you have concerns about your blood pressure or any other health-related issues, consult with your healthcare provider for personalized advice and guidance.

SUMMARY

"The Truth About Hypertension" is an informative and comprehensive book that delves into the complex world of high blood pressure, offering a detailed exploration of its causes, symptoms, and treatment options. With a focus on providing accurate and up-to-date information, this book aims to empower readers with the knowledge they need to understand and manage this prevalent health condition.

The book begins by demystifying the concept of hypertension, shedding light on its definition, prevalence, and the importance of blood pressure regulation. It takes the reader on a journey through the various risk factors that contribute to the development of high blood pressure, including genetics, lifestyle choices, and underlying medical conditions. By highlighting these factors, readers gain a deeper understanding of how hypertension can affect different individuals.

Understanding the symptoms of hypertension is crucial
for early detection and intervention. This book explores
the common signs and indicators of high blood
pressure, including persistent headaches, dizziness,
fatigue, and shortness of breath. By recognizing these
symptoms, readers are encouraged to seek timely
medical attention, potentially preventing the onset of
serious complications.

One of the book's key strengths lies in its detailed
examination of the treatment options available for
hypertension. It discusses both non-pharmacological
approaches and pharmaceutical interventions,
emphasizing the importance of lifestyle modifications
such as adopting a healthy diet, engaging in regular
exercise, and managing stress. Additionally, the book
explores the role of medication, highlighting different
classes of antihypertensive drugs and their mechanisms
of action.

"The Truth About Hypertension" recognizes that
managing high blood pressure requires a holistic
approach. It delves into the significance of regular

monitoring, self-care practices, and the value of a supportive healthcare team. By providing practical tips and guidance, the book equips readers with the tools needed to take control of their blood pressure and lead a healthier life.

Throughout the book, the author emphasizes the importance of patient education and empowerment. By dispelling common myths surrounding hypertension and presenting evidence-based information, readers are empowered to make informed decisions about their health. The book also addresses the potential complications that can arise from uncontrolled hypertension, such as heart disease, stroke, and kidney problems, further highlighting the urgency of managing this condition effectively.

In summary, "The Truth About Hypertension" serves as an invaluable resource for anyone seeking a comprehensive understanding of high blood pressure. With its insightful exploration of the causes, symptoms, and treatment options, this book aims to educate,

empower, and ultimately improve the lives of
individuals living with hypertension.

Printed in Great Britain
by Amazon

47041132R00106